Feeding Your Spirit
Food for the Soul

Eating & Living Holistically

By Reine Matthews

To those of you who want to lead healthier,
happier, more fulfilling lives.
This book is here to help you on that journey.

Blessings to all.

Table of Contents

Dear Reader,

This book is intended as an introduction to the holistic way of eating and living. How you use this book is up to you. I talk about why one would want to change to a holistic way of eating and living, then cover ways to transition from how you eat and live now to a more holistically based way of living and being. If making a life change is what you are going for, the first part of the book will be great for you.

This is also a cookbook, therefore, I know many of you will just want to use it for the recipes without reading the beginning and that's okay too. Whatever you take out of this book and how you use it will be right and good for you. So please enjoy. I thank you and bless you on your journey through the pages and trying the recipes, may you find health and healing as you transition to a more holistically balanced way of life and eating.

With love and gratitude,

Reine Matthews

Chapter 1

Introduction

What does it mean to feed your spirit? What is food for the soul? These are questions you might be wondering about as you pick up this book, and I am very glad you did. I will explain to you how to feed your spirit by eating the foods that will feed your soul. In doing so, you will feel lighter, healthier, and happier, which will create a more fulfilling life of well-being and vitality for you and your loved ones.

If you are looking for a new approach that isn't just about exercise and losing weight and is more about nourishing yourself in all ways, then this book is for you. When you feed your soul, you automatically feed your body in ways that heal, and both things together can ensure a long and happy life for you and your family.

We will begin by examining what food for the soul is. For starters, it is eating holistically, naturally, and simply. When you eat well, by putting natural foods into your body, your body will thank you and you will feel the difference. It's about eating mostly plant-based foods and getting away from processed food. You will notice how different it is when you eat well, by nourishing and feeding your body, vs. when you just fill it with artificial, chemical, and processed foods that give you the illusion of being full, but isn't actually giving you any real nutritional value. When you drop those false foods from your life, and put REAL food into your body, full of beneficial nutrients, that is when your body transforms on its own without you even realizing it.

You will lose weight, your skin will clear and glow, you will feel more energized, you will move easier, have fewer aches and pains, and so forth. That happened when I started changing my diet and way of life to a more holistically based way of being, I didn't even mean to lose weight, that wasn't even my intention, I just knew I needed to do something different, something that would help my body regain its strength and heal. And as I went forward on this journey the weight came off all on its own. Slowly I implemented new things and eliminating those "bad" things, no more refined sugars, no more processed foods, no more fast food of any kind. Slowly over time, I felt better and better. This didn't happen overnight, so please don't expect it to. Just know if I can do it, so can you. Doing just one change at a time. That is all it takes.

For me, the first thing I eliminated was processed foods. I stopped buying pre-made meals, or pre-packaged foods and stopped going to fast food restaurants out of convenience. I have always loved to cook and make things from scratch, however, even I would break down and go the "easy" route and have something pre-made from the store, or pick something up real quick at a drive-through. I finally concluded though that it wasn't doing me any good. So I started cooking more and more from scratch at home and often made enough to eat again the next day. That way if I didn't feel like cooking that next day I at least knew I had something good to eat that could be reheated later.

Next, I eliminated refined sugars. No more store-bought baked goods. No more homemade baked goods made the old fashioned traditional way. I researched and tried many things until I decided upon using coconut sugar in place of traditional white sugar. It bakes well and is an even equivalent to sugar in recipes, meaning that if a recipe calls for a ½ cup of sugar, you can use a ½ cup of coconut sugar in its place. Coconut sugar is low on the glycemic index so it doesn't spike your blood sugar levels as regular white sugar does, it also has retained some of its natural nutrients which white sugar does not have because of the intense processing that goes into making white refined sugar.

Gluten and wheat products were the next things to go. Now, this was a hard one at first because I loved bread and pasta. My favorite kind of food was Italian food, and I made pasta at home all the time, and loved freshly baked bread. My doctor actually recommended that I stop consuming gluten and see how I felt, and it made a difference for me, and honestly, this is when I noticed the weight come off me. No more bread of any kind, no more pasta. I ate much more veggies and finding other fun things to eat instead. Now even though this one took a while for me to stop altogether it was completely worth it. I not only released weight after this, but I had less digestive upsets and issues. So I must remind you to be gentle with yourself, and know it won't happen overnight. Just do the best you can. And know that it gets better and easier as you keep up with it. I rarely eat bread or wheat products anymore, except for the rare occasion of eating organic bread with a special meal. Nor do I eat any pasta, unless it's gluten free, and only for a rare special moment when I feel like making spaghetti or chicken marinara (which you can do without pasta and I often do now.) It is very rare for me to eat either thing even though I make sure it's organic or gluten-free. I must also point out that I tried many gluten-free bread and pasta and found that most were not quite the same, therefore, I decided I would rather just go without than try to eat an alternative and have it not be the same. That is why it's so rare for me to eat those things now. Once you eliminate them from your diet and keep it up for a while, you no longer have a desire to eat those foods, you no longer crave them or want them anymore. It's as if they don't exist in a way because you don't want or need them.

I encourage you to try gluten-free options and see for yourself if you like them or not, you may find you like some and that's fine if you do. For baking, I now use Namaste Foods Gluten Free All Purpose Flour Baking Blend. It is also free all the major food allergens. It tastes wonderful and makes great cookies. I use that with coconut sugar and it makes them that much better for you. I have also found that Udis Gluten Free bread is a good alternative to regular wheat bread if you like to eat sandwiches and such. Which has never been my thing even before going gluten-free. But it is an option to consider when going gluten-free. I must point out however even if you start cooking and baking gluten-free and use coconut sugar, you still must keep it at a minimum. You want to keep your sugar content low for your body. You want to make sure your liver can function at optimal capacity and sugars can hinder that if you do too much, even better choices like coconut sugar and other natural sweeteners like raw honey and organic maple syrup can still tax the body if overly consumed. So do your best to keep it at a minimum.

Some people have a hard time with grains, even gluten-free grains and that is where the use of almond flour and coconut flour come in. They are both great for certain things, but not everything. However, if you want to get away from all grains, which is highly beneficial for the digestive system, these are the best choices and I will supply recipes in the book that use them so you can try them and see how you like them. Keep an open mind and at least give these things a try.

Now that there has been an elimination of gluten and wheat in my diet, I also use gluten-free oats and oat bran, which I love. I even blend oats and almonds in a blender until a powder fine flour comes from it and make oat bran muffins with it in place of regular flour and it tastes great. Also using oat flour adds extra fiber to the diet that is most beneficial to the digestive system. You can also use almond meal flour on its own or with coconut flour to make it grain free, for some things. Experiment with these different things and discover what you like best. If you like bran muffins at all you will love the two recipes I have later in the book. I provide my favorite recipes here in the book to help you transition and most are gluten free and dairy free. I am giving you the information in this book to help you to decide what you feel is best for you and your family as far as diet goes. How far you want to go with it is your choice, but be willing to try them out.

Another very important thing I implemented while making these changes was juicing and making smoothies. Most people often do one or the other. They either do juicing and just drink the juice, or they make smoothies with milk or other base and just do smoothies, but I do things different. I juice certain fruits and veggies, usually the harder ones like root veggies and apples, and then use that juice as a base to then blend with more fruit and veggies for a nutrient-packed start to my day. I do it every day for breakfast and have done so for years. Ever since I started eating better and making these changes, juicing and smoothies have gone hand and hand with it all. I now do it every day as a habit for breakfast and will never go back to conventional breakfasts. It is a great way to start my day. You want to stick to the 20/80 rule, meaning 20 percent fruit and 80 percent veggies to keep the sugar content low.

As I was doing these things something happened within me, I felt more connected to my spirit than ever before, and I wanted more. My intuition opened up more, my connection to spirit, higher power, the universe (or whatever word you wish to use to describe it.) became stronger. And I started a healing journey, not just in healing my body, but also my mind, my emotions, and soul. I began with the healing of my body and gained so much more. I obtained the healing of my SELF. My whole SELF. Parts of me I didn't even know existed until I opened my heart and mind and it all slowly came to the surface. Grateful for the acknowledgment, my spirit helped me to heal the rest of myself, just as healing my body helped me to heal my spirit.

That is what I hope for you in reading this book. May you embark on a healing journey, of not only your body, but of your mind, your emotions, and your spirit. Healing your body starts with feeding it with the right foods that nourish and offer proper nutrition, healing your mind starts with paying attention to your mindset and finding ways to be more positive and see your life in positive ways, next it's always good to listen to your body emotionally. What I mean by that is how do you feel? What is your body telling you about how you feel? How does your body react to certain things? What might it be telling you about your emotional state? These are just some things to think about because later we'll dive into how to answer these questions and how to be open to feeling our feelings and allowing ourselves that space to express them in healthy ways. These things combined are what heals our spirit and nourishes our soul. Once all these things are in place you will then live from a place of holistic balance. And balance is what we all need in our lives today. So if you are ready, please read on and take that first step on your path, the journey to feeding your spirit with food for the soul.

Chapter 2

The Harm of Chemical, Processed, Artificial Food

Why are these things bad you might wonder and some results found in studies might shock you, but really to put it simply, the bottom line is this, these things are bad because they are not real food, I will say it again, they are NOT REAL FOOD. They don't provide proper nutrients, they provide things that the body can't even recognize as anything useful. Foods full of chemicals are overly processed, have additives in them, artificial flavorings, food dyes, GMOs (genetically modified organisms) which are harmful and do not nourish your body. They hold little to no nutritional value. They are merely fillers that give you the illusion of feeling full but don't actually give you anything that will properly fuel and heal your body.

Often the things added are substances like artificial vitamins and nutrients to make it look like it is good for you, but if it wasn't so highly processed, to begin with, they wouldn't have to add in artificial nutrients. Real food already has nutrients in it, naturally. The processing of foods often eliminates those nutrients, therefore, causing the food companies to add them back into the food with artificial vitamins and other nutrients. Wheat is one thing that is so highly processed these days that the bread companies have to add the B Vitamins back in once the flour has had those vital nutrients all processed out of it. White bread literally has no nutritional value, that is why it's white, all the natural nutrients in wheat have been processed out of it and made into a bread that's merely a filler and nothing more. This is just one basic example. There are so many other misleading things going on with our food system it is sad and scary. The best course of action is to learn these things and do your best to find and eat REAL foods, or SOUL foods, which I will go into later.

Right now I want to point out some disturbing evidence of the harm that can come from the Standard American Diet. Regarding food dyes, there are three widely used culprits—Yellow 5, Yellow 6 and Red 40— which all contain harmful compounds, including benzidine and 4-aminobiphenyl, that research has linked with cancer. Research also associates food dyes with health concerns and issues among children including allergies, hyperactivity, learning impairments, irritability and aggressiveness. I can tell you from experience as a young child in the '80s (yes even back then there were culprits) any time I had anything with red dyes in it I would puke it up and be sick for at least a day if not longer. My body was trying to get those toxins out of me to protect me from the harmful substance it was. I was basically suffering from a form of food poisoning, caused by red food dyes.

There are also many other additives and I will address some here and share their link to certain health problems. Nitrites, nitrates, artificial sweeteners, and the food dyes above are all linked to cancer. Sulfites often cause allergic reactions or aggravate asthma or even bring forth the onset of asthma. Sugars and sweeteners of all kinds are linked to candida overgrowth (yeast infections), diabetes, hypoglycemia, and obesity. Unfortunately, sugars are one of the most highly used additives in foods, especially processed food. It is also an inflammatory food, therefore if you already have inflammation in the body, such as arthritis or autoimmune diseases then sugars will just make those symptoms worse. Sugars are also highly addictive and often hard to eliminate from the diet without some really good self-control. MSG causes allergic reactions, headaches, dizziness, depression and mood swings, therefore if you already suffer from one or more of these ailments could it be that you are eating foods with this additive in it, making your symptoms worse, or could your symptoms be caused directly by this and other additives? The answer could be yes on both accounts, but it would be best to consult a doctor to know for sure. But ,this just shows it is possible your own health concerns could be aggravated or brought on by the food you eat if you consume these things regularly. Most of the U.S. Population consumes these things regularly and don't even think anything of it. Whether or not these additives are causing your symptoms, they will not help you heal or recover from these symptoms, the only way to do that is to eliminate them from your diet altogether and then see how you feel, you might be surprised.

Next is Gluten, some of you may know about this protein being an issue these days, it has become more and more common for people to want to eat gluten-free. What is gluten you might wonder, it is a protein found in wheat products. If it has wheat in it then it likely contains gluten. Barley and rye can also contain gluten, so be careful if you go gluten-free, there are lots of labels to be read to make sure there are no hidden forms of gluten in something. You can always look for certified Gluten Free foods, that way you know there will be no gluten contained. Why is gluten a problem? For some, if they have Celiac disease gluten causes them much hurt and basically destroys the digestive system. For those who are gluten sensitive it can do similar things internally but on a smaller scale. Gluten is also an inflammatory food, therefore causing and exacerbating inflammation in the body. For someone like myself who has dealt with an autoimmune disease personally, you want to stay away from inflammatory foods and eat anti-inflammatory foods instead to combat the effects of the dis-ease.

Dairy is another one, but it's kind of in a gray area for me. I have eliminated my consumption of dairy considerably and rarely eat any dairy anymore and when I do it's either organic butter or cheese. An even better choice with butter is Ghee basically clarified butter, meaning that the lactose and casein have been taken out of it making it easier for the body to digest. I consume no other dairy at all these days. Milk is difficult because it is so highly processed nowadays, therefore, you aren't actually getting milk in it's truest most natural form, which like bread as I mentioned earlier, just have the nutrients put back into it, artificially I might add, which makes it an unknown substance to the body. Dairy is also an inflammatory food, so that is why I keep my use of it to the bare bones minimum. Dairy is often hard for people to get away from, especially cheese. Cheese (and other dairy products) contain casein, which is also an addictive substance, much like sugar. Another point about dairy is that cows are often injected with hormones and other such things that cause their milk to contain those same compounds which we don't need in our bodies. The last thing we need to do is consume extra hormones, especially artificial ones. If you want to keep dairy around in your diet, I would highly recommend buying only that which is organic, from cows that are hormone free and grass fed, and only consume it on an occasional basis. Raw cultured dairy is an even better option. Making sure it still contains all the beneficial probiotics in it ensures that it will help instead of hinder your body. Raw cheese, raw fresh milk straight from the cow, and raw cultured plain yogurt are all good choices. Goats milk is also a great choice since it is tolerated much better than cow dairy. Goats milk kefir is something everyone should have regularly to heal the gut and provide more of those great probiotics that help with digestion. I will go into more detail in another chapter on gut healing foods. Goat cheese is a better cheese choice too, also get it raw if you can. Goats milk is easily tolerated and does not cause any adverse effects like cows milk often does. That is because it is more like human breast milk in its makeup than cows milk. It is also less likely to be processed like cows milk because there aren't as many people making goats milk. Again with all these options keep the intake at a minimum, but at least there are options. There are dairy free options too, I would stick to almond, cashew, or coconut milk products that have little to no sugars added and you're good to go there. But check the labels and make sure there aren't a lot of fillers and things added to it. Sometimes a lot of things still are added instead of keeping it simple and most natural. We all have to watch out for our food and discover what's really in it to make sure it's natural and good for our bodies.

GMOs are genetically modified organisms. What that means is that the GMO foods are usually made in a lab first, then grown. Which is unnatural. Using GMOs is rampant and disturbing. Most were RoundUp Ready, so the food itself contains Round Up, compounds that kill off bugs automatically when a bug lands on it. So if it kills bugs who touch this food and/or eats this food, what do you think is happening to your insides when you consume this food? Watch the documentary "FOOD MATTERS" to discover more in-depth information on the subject. I know people might say something like "but a bug is so much smaller than us, how can it hurt us?" Well eating these genetically modified foods over time can cause a world of hurt. Especially in the digestive system where it wreaks havoc. GMOs basically destroy the digestive system slowly. So you won't have symptoms of any kind for a long time, but then you will realize that you cannot eat certain foods, that your body isn't digesting like it used to, and some things make you sick that never did before. GMOs do that, it takes its time and destroys the body from the inside out. You really must pay attention to your food and make sure none of it is genetically modified. GMOs have been linked to the possible cause of gluten intolerance and celiac disease, cancer, the onset of so many autistic children, learning difficulties, ADD and ADHD and more. You see when your body isn't being nourished properly with real natural food, it causes disruptions in the body expressed in multiple different forms. Do your research, look these things up online, watch documentaries like "Food Matters" and get educated on these things to understand what's going on with our food supply. Knowledge is the best way to ensure you eat well and nourish your body and your family properly.

     If you haven't noticed the trend here yet, all these things are causing our foods to become unrecognizable by our bodies as food and our body has a hard time breaking it down, or even using it for anything other than the illusion of being full. Many things are destroying the basic bodily functions, causing problems with digestion, which can cause so many illnesses and diseases. The digestive system is important to the ability of the immune system to work properly, so if your digestive system becomes out of balance or unable to function as it should, the immune system slowly fails, and the body develops dis-ease and illness. If we want to take precautionary measures and do what we can to prevent these things in the first place, it would be best to eliminate all these things and only put real food into the body. Food that is nutritious, gives the body the proper nutrients it needs to function well, and food that feeds the soul.

Chapter 3

Eating SOUL Foods

SOUL foods come down to this, Seasonal, Organic, Unprocessed, and Local. Which means you want to try your best to eat food in season, one reason for this is that in season foods usually costs less because it's their peak time to be available, it is also often a great way to easily get produce. You want organic food to ensure that it is as close to its natural form as possible as if it were just freshly picked, and if you grow your own food that makes it that much better and that much fresher. The fresher the food and the closer it is to its natural state, the more nutrients it holds within. Therefore, it's much better for you, giving you the best nutrition possible. Unprocessed is very important since the processing of foods breaks down and often depletes the nutritional value of the foods and often they become nothing more than just a filler with no nutritional value left. Not only that, but processed foods often contain loads of chemicals and additives never meant for the body to ingest or break down, and sometimes the body can't break them down and it can cause upset and disease in the body because of it, along with other harmful effects of chemicals and additives. If it's not naturally derived then you shouldn't put it in your body. Local comes in to prevent the carbon footprint of your food. The longer it takes to get to you or your grocery store the more time, energy, and fuel is being used. If you buy local food you are not only limiting the carbon footprint, you are also supporting local growers and local businesses, which boots the local economy and helps your neighbors. Another thing to point out about local is that the food is likely to be fresher because it doesn't take as long to get to you as imported foods or foods from other parts of the country. Earlier the fresher the food, the more nutrients it carries, and the better it is for you and your family to eat and fuel yourselves.

How to eat seasonal foods: seasonalfoodguide.org is a great place to start. It is an interactive website where you put in your location and the month and it will tell you what foods are in season for your area at any specified time of year. This will help you get educated on what is in season near you and what to look out for and when. Also while shopping most produce in season is usually in abundance and at a better price than others because they are in season. You can also create recipes for each season that utilizes the produce that is ready and in abundance for those times of the year. That way you are prepared when that season comes around each year. It may take some time, learning, and planning, but once you have it all figured out and set up, you will be set for years to come. So it may seem like a lot of work at first, just know that it will have long term benefits in the end.

Eating Organic: This one is self-explanatory and easy to start right away. Just look for foods labeled as organic. Buy organic produce, and as much other food items labeled organic and certified gluten-free if you go that route. There are higher standards and more rules regarding the growing and creating of organic food so they are labeled well. Labels to look for are certified gluten-free labels and USDA Organic. The one thing I will point out about organic foods is that you still need to be careful of pre-made, pre-packed, and somewhat processed organic foods, they often still have a lot of added sugars and other fillers that you may not want to consume. Getting into the habit of always checking labels is crucial. Get to know what is in your food and if there are things you don't recognize on the label you may want to reconsider if it's something you want to consume or not. Organic is better, but with things like cereals, crackers, breads, chips, and other pre-packed foods they can still have some additives and/or a lot more sugar than you should be consuming. Just be aware of that and keep it in mind as you learn to transition.

Going Unprocessed: This one might be harder at first, but it is well worth it. Stop buying boxed foods, pre-made meals, anything with additives, preservatives, and food dyes. This requires reading labels, however, if you start to just buy organic and avoid buying anything that is not labeled organic this process becomes much easier since most organic foods are minimally processed if at all. They also don't contain additives or chemical preservatives or harmful food dyes. That is another reason going organic is so much easier and so much better for you. It makes the switch to unprocessed food a snap, since all you then have to do is look for certified organic food, and it eliminates all the bad stuff in one easy step. Another great and easy way to stay unprocessed is to buy mainly produce and start cooking for yourself. You want to eat mostly plant-based foods anyway to ensure that you are getting enough nutrients in your diet. If you don't know how to cook, then this is a great time to learn. Also, there are many whole foods you can eat easily without even knowing how to cook. Such as salads, you have only to put a salad mix in a bowl and add dressing, or a fruit bowl you can just chop fruit and put in a bowl with nuts and coconut yogurt and you're done. Plus pretty much any produce item you can just pick up, clean it, and eat it right then and there as is. There are many more things just like I will have in the recipe part of this book along with other recipes that require more cooking. So you can go for more in-depth recipes or go the easy route with little to no cooking involved, but still be able to eat well.

Another thing to know with unprocessed foods is animal products, mainly meat, dairy, and eggs. There has to be processing of these things to be able to have it available in stores for people buy it and use it, however, there are things to look for regarding meat, dairy, and eggs. The things to be mindful of is what has been done to it. You want to find hormone free, free range, and grass fed. You may also eliminate meat from your diet, and you can if you like, but for those who still plan to eat meat, these are the best options for you regarding animal-based food items. Do what is right for you. Eating vegan and vegetarian are not for everyone, so try different things and discover how your body responds and eat. Some people do well by eliminating animal products and others do not. Just know that even if it works great for others doesn't mean it's right for you and even if it works great for you, doesn't mean it's good for everyone else. We are all different in our make-up, therefore, we will all respond differently to different things and that is why it's important to know what your body likes and doesn't like, to notice how it feels after eating certain things, eat what makes you feel good inside and eliminate what makes you feel yucky inside. That is part of noticing how you are feeling, notice how you feel after you eat, do you feel energized and well nourished? Or do you feel drained, tired, and sluggish? That will show you what is good for you or what is not so good for you and then you can start to eat in a way that makes you feel good.

Buying Local: This may take some research if you aren't already in the know about your local food offerings. Search for farmer's markets in your area, roadside food stands from local growers and farmers, local health food stores if you have one or more, find as much information about the nearest farmers and what they grow, other growers nearby, co-ops, markets, you-pick farms, and more. If you haven't already, you could go to a you-pick farm and you will be in for a treat. That is when you go to the farm itself and pick your own produce from whatever they have available at the time and in season. Therefore you are not only eating local but seasonally. Once you find all these things, go and check them out in person, get to know your local growers, find the things you like that they offer and support local business simultaneously.

Also as a side note I have labeled certain recipes as vegan for those who may want to try eating vegan, or for anyone who is already vegan who wants to try some of these recipes and it's just a quick way to know which one's most certainly are okay for vegans. It also just means that those recipes are dairy-free, meat-free, and free of any animal products. It does not mean that non-vegans can't eat them, it's just an easy way to find recipes that are free of animal-based ingredients. You can eat any of these recipes as you choose so don't let the labels make you think otherwise. If it sounds good try it.

Chapter 4

Gut Healing Foods

Many of us have compromised immune systems and damaged digestive systems and we don't even know it. The gut is one of the most important parts of the immune system, therefore if there is damage in the digestive system, there will be a weakened immune system. Hippocrates, the father of modern medicine, stated that "All disease begins in the gut." Think about that for a moment, there is no surprise that people dealing with health issues also have gut and digestive issues along with it. The standard American diet, consisting of high sugar, GMOs, processing, and food dyes, just exacerbates these imbalances and issues. Not to mention they often can cause these issues as well. It is the point of this book to help heal those imbalances. One of the best ways to do that is to incorporate gut healing foods into your diet.

What are gut healing foods? Foods high in micro-nutrients and macro-nutrients, foods loaded with naturally occurring probiotics and prebiotics, foods easy for the body to digest, and repair the gut lining.

The number one gut healing food is bone broth. Making bone broth at home is easy and the best way to get the beneficial nutrients this stuff carries. It is full of collagen, which helps heal the gut lining and the skin. It is also good for joints and other connective tissue in the body. It contains all the essential amino acids our body needs to function. It is one of the most nutrient dense "light" foods out there. What I mean by a "light" food is that it is low in calories and easy for the body to digest and use. The collagen and the abundance of nutrients and amino acids it contains is what makes it the best food for healing the gut.

Probiotic-rich foods are another group of foods great for healing the gut. Foods like kefir, raw cultured dairy, unsweetened plain yogurt, sauerkraut, kimchi, and other fermented veggies all contain probiotics and some prebiotics. Which help to heal the gut and keep it in balance. That is what holistic eating is all about, maintaining balance within the body through diet and lifestyle. In the case of sauerkraut and other fermented foods you want to make sure they are made with just the produce itself and water. You don't want to use ones made with vinegar or have additives in them. Those can actually hurt your internal system which is the opposite of what we want to do when consuming gut healing foods.

Other gut healing foods are aloe vera juice, coconut, steamed or boiled veggies, ginger, and blueberries. Aloe vera juice is very soothing and healing to the digestive tract. It contains antioxidants, enzymes, minerals, and fatty acids. It normalizes the acid-alkaline balance in the body and is anti-inflammatory. Coconut is anti-viral, anti-bacterial, and anti-fungal, it contains healthy fats, it has anti-inflammatory and analgesic properties, it destroys bad bacteria and candida. Which make it a powerhouse for healing. Steamed or boiled vegetables are easy for the body to digest and contain lots of vitamins and nutrients and fiber that help keep the flow of elimination. Ginger is a great tonic for the stomach and digestive system. It helps to relax the GI tract, it can kill harmful bacteria in the body, and helps you absorb more nutrients. Blueberries help heal the digestive system with its antioxidants and fiber content, while also being anti-inflammatory.

Once you eliminate all the harmful foods mentioned in an earlier chapter, do a bone broth fast to cleanse your digestive system before eating holistically if you need that drastic of a change. Some people will need it more than others and it is up to you if you do one. Even if you choose not to do a fast, you would benefit from adding all these foods into your diet. It must be done slowly to not shock your system because that could cause more harm than good. Especially if you incorporate fermented probiotic-rich foods and your body is not used to having them, you will want to add them into your diet in slow increments. Like doing one teaspoon of one fermented food a day for about a week, and then moving up to take one tablespoon of one fermented food a day, then you can eat them more than once a day, but still do only one tablespoon of each to start, and build upon that as you go. See how your body feels and reacts, it will tell you if it's too much too soon, so back it off if that occurs.

It's important to incorporate these foods into your diet for an overall sense of health and well-being. To create balance in your system and heal your gut in whatever capacity is needed for your individual needs. Check out my blog www.reinematthews.com/blog for more details on doing a bone broth fast, and the elimination diet I did prior to fasting and slowly incorporating foods back into your diet after the fast. I posted how I prepared for the fast, how I did the fast and what I experienced, and then how I slowly added foods back into my diet once the fast was over. So check it out if you want more information about fasting with bone broth.

One more thing to consider regarding foods that are easier for the body to digest is soaking nuts and seeds before using them and eating them. The importance of soaking nuts and seeds is to make them more bio-available, to reduce the lectins, and make them easier for the body to process.

Being more bio-available is the higher degree to which the food's nutrients are available for absorption and utilization in the body. Eating food highly available, making it better utilized by the body, the greater the benefit you get from what you are eating. The more nutrients you get in your diet the better your body will feel and the better it will function. That's why it's great to incorporate foods in a way that make them more bio-available.

Lectins are plant proteins that bind to certain sugars causing agglutination. This can cause blood cells to clump and may have negative effects on our cells and blood system depending on what is causing the agglutination. These negative effects can wreak havoc on the internal systems of the body. These proteins are basically the plant's protection against predators, meaning it has an attacking function, therefore you don't want something in your system that would have the function of attack. Lectins are found mostly in nuts and seeds of most if not all vegetables and fruits.

I am not an expert on lectins, I am just learning about them, but what little I have come across made me feel the need to add it to this book for basic reference. You may research it more yourself to get a better idea of what they are and how they affect the body. I just know that soaking nuts and seeds makes them easier for the body to process and use and that makes the body happy. Therefore it's just something I would like you all to consider regarding eating healthy and gaining overall wellness. Most especially for those who know they have a compromised digestive system or poor gut health.

Chapter 5

Blessings, Gratitude, and Food

Did you know that blessing your food and expressing gratitude for your food, can enhance the eating experience, and bring forth good vibes to your food and to your body once you eat that food? I know this may seem far fetched at first, but blessing your food actually can enhance your food. How does it do this? Well, there have been many studies about how positive words affect water and can actually heal contaminated water, so the same thing holds true with our food and our bodies. Most produce and our bodies consist of mostly water, so if words affect water, it will also affect us personally and the food we eat. If we speak positive loving words over our food, which blessings are, it will enhance the nutrients and the positive life force of that food. When we then eat that food, our bodies are absorbing those good vibes and life force, and that keeps the body strong and healthy. It is sad to see how saying grace before meals have gone by the wayside these days because it was a positive thing for our food and our bodies. Don't do it in a traditional sense if you are not religious in any way, you can just say something like, "I am grateful for this food I am about to eat and I thank it for it's healing properties and nutrients that nourish my body." That alone will do wonders for your eating experience and lift your spirits and make you feel good. Especially when done over time you will be amazed at how great it feels and the effects it will have on your overall well-being.

Gratitude is a form of prayer, but it need not be done in prayer form to be beneficial. Expressing gratitude is good for all of us, it helps us to have a more positive outlook on life, to have an overall sense of well-being, and brings forth a more positive mindset as the practice is continued. Expressing gratitude for our food and what it can do for us is a great way to enhance mealtime, and bring forth a feeling of appreciation for what you are doing for yourself and that includes eating well. As we take care of ourselves and express gratitude for those things, we feel better about ourselves and our lives. Our bodies will thank us for it.

If you grow your own food or keep a garden of any kind, blessing the garden and expressing gratitude for what you are growing can have added benefits and enhancements to your food and what you are growing. There have been studies done that show when plants are spoken to with kind positive words they grow better. What better way to have a garden than one that grows well with abundance because you had only to speak kindly and positively to it and express your gratitude for its growth. It's amazing what the right words and attitude can do for our lives, including the lives of plants, whether you eat them or not. To have an abundant garden, speak kindly and positively to it and express love and gratitude for it and see how it thrives and grows. Do you notice how good you feel when you speak kindly and positively to yourself? Do you notice how good it feels when someone offers you a compliment or expresses gratitude for you or something you have done? Those same effects can happen to all living things, plants, animals, and food included.

That is why blessing your food is so beneficial. Whether it's still growing in the garden, or ready to eat on your table, bless it, express gratitude for it, and what it provides for you, and great things will come of it. Notice how good you feel too while you are doing it, it's good for all things. So why not do it? It's so easy, practice it and over time you can make it a new habit. One that will reap benefits for years to come and pass it on to your children and grandchildren so they too may reap the rewards of good vibes, and food for the soul.

When blessing your food and offering gratitude, you are not only benefiting your meal, you are feeding your soul. You are connecting to your higher self and the divine. Whatever it may be for you, (God, Spirit, Universe, and so forth) don't get too caught up in what words to use, or how to express it, make it simple so it works best for you, it is all effective either way. As long as your intentions are positive and good, you can't go wrong.

What all this has to do with is energy, the energy you put out and the energy you are putting into your body through the food you eat.

Everything is energy, however, since all things are energy, all words carry energy. Thoughts also carry energy. Words and thoughts can carry either negative or positive energy. Obviously, positive energy will cause positive things and negative energy results in negative things. That is often how energy works. All living things are affected by energy, therefore, all living things are affected by words and thoughts, since they too are a form of energy. Negative words and thoughts can cause detrimental effects like depression, illness, and dis-ease, positive words and thoughts can bring forth healing and restorative effects like finding peace within and recovering from illness or dis-ease.

This also relates to our food, not only is food energy but since it is living before we harvest it and eat it, it is also affected by the energy directed towards it. What you say over your food can have positive or negative effects of that food before we even put it in our bodies. That is one reason saying "grace" before a meal is good practice to get into. Now it need not be religious if that is not your thing, all you basically need to do is express gratitude for the food, for it's nourishing and nurturing properties and for its ability to keep you strong, healthy, and help you heal if you need that. Thank your food for what it provides for you and thank it for providing that. This is most beneficial for those who garden and grow their own food. Go out and thank your food while it's still growing in the garden. Thank the plants for what they provide for you and your family. You will gain an abundance from doing this one little practice. You may be surprised at how much more things will thrive and grow in your garden when you do. Gratitude creates abundance and it works for all areas of life, not just food and eating.

The energy concept goes for what kind of food you are putting into your body. If the food you eat is still very much alive and full of energy, as in plants, containing living nutrients it will be much more beneficial for you than eating highly processed food that has had the life processed out of it and no longer contains any life force left to nourish you from the inside out. That is another reason eating organic, unprocessed foods is so important. That is also why eating mostly plant-based foods is so beneficial to the body and the healing process. You are what you eat, and when you put life force, energetic food into your body, your body will then contain the life force needed to heal or stay healthy and be strong and able to take you wherever you want to go in life.

Chapter 6

Is that hunger?
What are you really feeling?

Noticing how you feel before you eat, when you eat, and most after you eat is an important step in the process of transitioning to a holistically based lifestyle. Noticing how you feel before you eat can help you determine if you have times of emotional eating, so you can change the habit. Is it hunger that you are feeling or are you wanting to eat for some other reason? Emotional eating is when we eat because we are suppressing or stuffing down emotions we don't want to deal with, which could be loneliness, depression, anger, fear, insecurities, and more. Emotional eating often causes excessive weight gain and low self esteem. That is why it's important to discover if you suffer from emotional eating. I used to suffer from emotional eating, craving bread, cheese, and sugary sweets. I would often eat out of boredom or loneliness. I no longer have these urges anymore since changing my diet and eating holistically.

Noticing how you feel while you are eating can tell you quite a lot. Are you enjoying your meal, or are you eating quickly just to get it over with? Do you taste your food, or do you eat just because you know you need to eat? Do you feel good when you eat or are you feeling some other emotion? Do you like food? Do you like eating? Or do you feel negative emotions towards it? Pay attention to what is going on inside yourself. It will tell you a lot about yourself. It will also help you to figure out what exactly you like with food and eating and what are those things you genuinely dislike and would rather not eat. It's all okay.

How do you feel after you eat? What do certain foods do to you? Do you feel indigestion, do you have gas, is there bloating, do you feel constipated or do you have diarrhea? Genuinely notice and learn of how you feel when you eat certain foods. Notice when you feel good and energized after eating, and when you feel lethargic and sluggish. This will tell you a lot about your digestive system, what kind of state it may be in, and what foods to avoid, and the foods that make you feel good and should be consumed more often.

Start keeping a food diary to help you through this process if you wish. Write down everything you eat, when you eat, like what you had for breakfast, then how you felt later after eating, then lunch, and so forth, also add in any snacks throughout the day and notice how you feel after those. Then as you adjust your diet notice how things change, notice when you feel better and notice if you feel worse. Pay attention to what may be causing these things for you, the good and the bad. So you can find the best foods for your body.

This is all part of the learning process and the transition. You cannot switch over to a holistic way of doing anything without some transition and transformation. Because going holistic means merging all aspects of yourself, the physical, the emotional, the mental, and the spiritual. You cannot have one without the other, but many people run off of one or two and neglect the rest, but for eating and living holistically, you neglect none of them. You must connect and merge them all into a balanced state of being, so you may be a balanced being yourself. That is why contacting your feelings is part of the process. Why you need to discover what your present relationship with food and eating is so you can heal anything to be healed regarding mindset and emotions. So you can find a healthy connection to food and eating. That is also why blessings and prayer are important too, to cover the spiritual aspect of the human and ,eating right benefits the physical. Which bring all four aspects together as one healthy being when all pieces are put together.

Do you know what part of you is being neglected? Is it the physical, emotional, mental, or spiritual? In what ways are you functioning in life? Are you a go, go, go, type person who feels the need to be physically moving all the time? Then you focus on the physical more. Or are you constantly on the go due to stress and anxiety, worried about getting things done? That is mental and physical. Are you ruled by your emotions? Have you been called overly sensitive or overly emotional? Then you likely need to balance that with the other aspects because you are focusing on the emotional. How spiritual are you? Do you have any spiritual connection or practice? If you don't then that is a part of you that needs some cultivating to balance out the rest. Do you see how these examples make sense and how they can tie into each other? Or on the flip side are you too spiritual and neglect the rest of yourself by focusing on only spiritual things? There must be balance to have harmony in the body and in your life. If you focus too much on one or two parts and neglect the others then harmony will be lost, that is where imbalance starts and dis-ease can come forth. Learning about yourself in these ways can help you find health and wellness in ways you never thought possible before now.

Noticing how you feel about everything in life, about what you are doing and how you do it, feeling your body and noticing your internal systems, and figuring out where you are at within, so you can balance it and be better off inside and out. When you heal your inner life, your outer naturally gets better. As you focus on all aspects and become more positive and mindful, the outer world becomes a better and happier place. With balance and harmony comes an awareness of life and the world around you you weren't able to see before, and now with these changes, you can and you feel so much better for it. I know it may sound weird right now if you haven't made the changes yet and haven't paid attention, but once you do these things will come about and you will understand. Keep an open mind and an open heart as you read on and implement the things in this book.

Chapter 7

Mindset

Now you have discovered how you feel about food and eating and how eating certain foods make you feel, you can switch your mindset to a more positive one regarding food, eating, and life in general. If you find you have negative emotions regarding food and eating this is a great practice to start. Even if you have no negative thoughts or feelings towards food you can still implement this positive mindset towards eating and the holistic lifestyle. It will help with the transition and get you through the moments that feel hard to do.

Being grateful for the food and eating well is a wonderful start and that is why I spoke earlier about blessing your food and expressing gratitude. Taking it a step further, you can think about food as a wonderful amazing thing that helps your body, heals your body, and nourishes your body. Eating the right foods makes it possible for you to have energy, to feel good physically, to keep going every day, and function properly.

Having a healthy mindset around food and eating is just as important as eating healthy food. What were you taught to believe about eating and food as a child? Think back, was food and eating good, or was it made to be "bad" such as getting picked on for eating too much or too little or being overweight or underweight. Or were you allowed to eat well, any time you felt hungry, and enjoy your food. These things will come into play in your adult life and if you had negative experiences as a child around food then you might also have similar experiences with food as an adult you may want to heal to get to a place where food and eating are good and enjoyable parts of life.

There have been studies that show when children are restricted from food as a child they are more likely to overeat and indulge in unhealthy food as an adult. If a child is picked on regarding food, weight, or how they eat, it will affect their relationship with food, themselves, and others as an adult. You can see how all these things can affect the way you see food, feel about food, and how you approach eating in general. This is also important to know if you have children of your own and want to teach them how to eat well and have a positive relationship with food and eating themselves.

Start to see food as sacred, treat eating as a special ritual for health and vitality. Don't get elaborate with it either, it just comes down to mindset. Believe that food will heal, that food is nourishing, that eating is a good and beneficial part of life, that it will do great things for you. Even if you had a less than positive outlook on it as a child, which inhibited your relationship with food as an adult. Let that go, leave it in the past as best as you can to open yourself up to a new way to see and connect with food.

Don't be wasteful with food either. Use the food, try not to throw it out, unless it's unhealthy and bad for you or if it has gone bad. That way you can appreciate food and value it for what it is. It is natures way of nurturing, healing, and helping the body. Food makes the body able to function at full capacity and feel good and energized. That is when you eat the right foods. Harmful foods will have the opposite effect.

Start eating healthier more nutrient-rich foods and thank it for what it can do for you and your family. Teach your children, if you have any, the importance of food, and help them to have a happy, healthy experience with food and eating, so they can grow into a healthy happy adult.

What are positive things you can think of right now that you can honestly say about food? What are positive happy experiences you have had regarding eating? What do you enjoy about eating? What do you dislike? Get to know yourself and your eating preferences. Ask yourself these questions and focus on the good things and add to it as you go along. Here is an example:

Food is good it provides me with nourishment and the nutrients my body needs to heal, food tastes good, I enjoy food, I like eating fresh berries, they taste so sweet and juicy. My favorite kind of food is Mexican food. One of my favorite food experiences is when I had a bonfire for my birthday and my parents had a pot of chili on the wood stove and a pot of potato soup on the kitchen stove, it smelled wonderful and tasted so good, all my friends enjoyed it. Another favorite experience of food for me was more recent, I was taken out to dinner at an Organic restaurant, each meal was fabulous, they had this vegan carrot cake to die for, I am not even vegan, but it was so good, it was the best carrot cake I have ever had. I loved that night out and the food was the main event. We shared a vegetarian appetizer, we had organic bread with olive oil and balsamic, I had the duck and he had the chicken, then we shared that carrot cake, it was all wonderful quality tasting food, that was prepared with love. It is now my new favorite restaurant.

I love broccoli, I have since I was a kid, and that is good for me. Therefore I still eat broccoli today. My new favorite thing right now is Brussels sprouts and shallots. I had never eaten either until we went to that organic restaurant I mentioned before, now they are my two favorite things to eat together. I just loved how they made them and keep eating them now at home. See how these positive food experiences have enhanced my eating and my relationship with food?

To have an experience like that with food brings forth the desire to have more enjoyable experiences for eating. Those are just examples of how I would answer those questions right now at this moment. You can see how positive and empowering those words are and how good it feels to read them. Just reading that brings forth happy thoughts about food and eating.

I want That for you. I would like you to find that place in yourself where food is good, eating is enjoyable, and finding healthy choices is a new found passion of joy and excitement just as it has become for me. Even if you already enjoy food and eating, you can enhance it even more as you make healthier choices. You can celebrate those choices and accomplishments by making these changes and honoring yourself.

Chapter 8

Juicing & Smoothies

What is the difference between juicing and smoothies? Well, the obvious difference is that one takes fruits and veggies and reduces them down to the juice, and the other takes them and makes them into a more solid puree that contains all the fibers still in them. The juice no longer has the fiber content because it's just liquid. Juicing creates a more concentrated form of the nutrients quickly absorbed by the body, whereas a smoothie is slowly digested and contains more fiber important for the digestive system and preventing an insulin spike in your blood sugar levels. Because the juice has no fiber it is basically all sugars and can spike blood sugar levels, especially if it is made of mostly fruits. Therefore combining the two as I do to make my morning smoothie contains concentrated nutrients from the juice and added fiber from the solid fruits and veggies blended in to make a nutrient-packed powerhouse of a breakfast to start your day. It's also easy to do and take on the go if needed.

There are many options out there when you do juicing or smoothies, or both. The choice is up to you and depends on your lifestyle and how much time you will put into your breakfast. Juicing takes up a little more time than a straight up a smoothie, and combining the two adds a little more time, but it is well worth it if you will do it. Investing the time in yourself and your health is important, but I understand that people have busy lives and tend to be on the go to get it all done. So choose for yourself what you feel would work best for you.

The quickest and easiest is to make a basic smoothie. All you need is a good blender, a liquid such as almond milk, soy milk, coconut milk, coconut water or plain filtered water, and fruits and veggies you would like to blend. For blending some of the harder fruits and veggies may not be the best choice for they won't blend all the way and leave your smoothie chunky and hard to get down. Some of my favorite choices for a smoothie are all berries, pineapple, cucumber, zucchini, salad greens, kale, oranges, lemons, limes, celery, and so forth. Try your best to use more veggies than fruit to keep the sugar content low and the fiber content high. Experiment with different flavor combinations and find what you like best. Some people use ice, but I don't. Mainly because I use frozen berries I don't feel the need to use ice, plus ice makes it too cold for me. The choice is yours.

Juicing is easy as long as you have an actual juicer to use. Many of these high powered blenders these days are advertising themselves as a juicer, but it is different. You need an actual juicer to make juices, not a high powered blender. Though having a high powered blender comes in handy for a smoothie. Once you have an actual juicer you may proceed. You can juice most any fruit or vegetable. Read your owners manual for details on how the fruit and veggies should be prepped before juicing. Some want you to remove peels from oranges, lemons, limes, and other thick peals. Some suggest you use smaller pieces instead of whole, and so forth, but once you understand how your particular juicer works you can literally juice just about everything you want. Again more veggies than fruit is a good rule of thumb for the same reason as smoothies. Keep the sugar content lower. Certain things that should not be juiced because they don't have enough water content for juicing would be avocados, bananas, and potatoes. They would just make a huge nasty mess in your juicer.

Either practice will bring more nutrients into your body in which your body will thank you for. You will feel more energized and light, you won't be so bogged down or foggy. Making juices and smoothies jump starts your ability to function well and jump starts your immune system.

Now let's combine the two together, choose hard fruits and veggies to juice first. I mostly use zucchini, carrots, celery, ginger root, and apples. You could also use beets, broccoli, cabbage, cucumbers, and tomatoes. I also often juice my citrus as well because I am not a fan of pulp. So you can choose to juice citrus for less pulp, or blend them when you blend the smoothie and have the pulp, then you'll get more fiber so remember that. Put the juice into a blender and add frozen kale and frozen fruit like mixed berries, mangoes, or pineapple. You can choose any frozen fruit you like, I choose berries mostly for their fiber content, and low glycemic index rating, meaning they naturally have a lower sugar content, and I just love berries. I also add in supplements that you can do or not. You don't have to, for me, it just gives me that added pack of nutrients to start the day with. For me personally, I add in a tablespoon of flax seeds, a tablespoon of sunflower lecithin, a scoop of magnesium powder,, and sometimes vitamin C powder if I feel the need for it to boost the immune system like during cold and flu season. I also use pea protein powder. Pea protein is a good neutral tasting protein that is easier on the digestive system and is easily tolerated by most people. So it's a great choice for anyone, unless you are allergic to peas which is quite rare.

As you can see there are endless options of how you can approach juicing and making smoothies, there are also many options of combining fruits and veggies to your liking, and making it individually something for you to like and enjoy knowing it is good for you and will help your body in a multitude of ways. Again this is a great place to experiment and try different flavors and combinations. Enjoy your food and your creating with food. Creativity abounds with juicing and smoothies.

Also you can do either or both and throughout your day. It's not just for breakfast. You can make fresh juice to drink with a meal if you like, or have a smoothie as a quick snack or meal replacement later in the day. You could live off of juicing and smoothies if you like, but for me personally that would get old after a while, but you could do it and it would be good for the body, as long as you added in protein powder or nuts and seeds to ensure you get a balance amount of nutritional needs met.

If you didn't know or hadn't thought about it yes you can add in nuts, seeds, oats, and other odds and ends to your smoothies. Protein powder also comes in handy for an extra boost, and if you eat little meat, or go vegetarian or vegan it's imperative. Other things you can add in that you may not have thought about are chia seeds, avocados, coconut oil, hemp seeds, cacao powder, spirulina, acai powder, maca powder, matcha green tea powder for those of you who need a little boost of caffeine to start the day, cinnamon, and other spices.

So go out and get you a nice blender and a juicer if you choose and create, get in the kitchen and have fun with it. If you have kids involve them, they will have fun with it too and get creative themselves. It's great for the whole family, it brings you together and gets you all eating well and being healthy. That's something to celebrate. Grab a glass of fresh juice or a smoothie and toast to good health and a happy family.

Chapter 9

Simple Easy Meals

Great simple meals you can create yourself with little to no cooking involved, these include salads, soups, stews, and veggie dishes. This chapter is for those of you who either have no cooking experience, are just learning how to prepare meals, or want something quick and easy who are strapped for time.

Salads: greens, veggies, and fruit tossed together. Easy peasy.
Salad Basics:
Mixed salad greens you can buy in the store already together.
Or a combination of lettuce and greens of any kind, such as:
romaine, red leaf, chard, kale, arugula, iceberg, spinach, bib, loose leaf.
Sliced fruit:
apples, pineapple, all berries, pears, mangoes
Nuts and seeds:
walnuts, pecans, almonds, pumpkin seeds, macadamia nuts, hemp seeds
Veggies: sliced carrots, zucchini, cucumber, broccoli, cauliflower, olives, beets, Brussels sprouts, cabbage, peas, and more.
Beans: Black beans, lima beans, red beans, kidney beans, pinto beans, chickpeas, and white beans.

You need only to toss any variation of these items together in a bowl, add dressing and you're ready to eat my friend. I would suggest buying organic salad dressings that are dairy free, or you can make your own which is easy. The most basic homemade dressing is 1/3 cup of olive oil, 1 tablespoon of apple cider vinegar, the juice of half a lemon, and salt and pepper. Put in a small jar, shake and serve. I have recipes for other salad dressing variations in the recipe section.

You can also make a fruit salad by adding any variation of sliced fruits with berries, nuts and seeds, and lemon juice, toss together and you have yourself an easy and healthy fruit salad.

One other kind of salad you can do is a bean salad. Take multiple types of cooked or canned beans and toss together, add dressing, and there you have it.

I don't have too many recipes in the book for salads because they are so easy to make, can be very individual for each person making them, and so I am just giving you the basics you need to start creating salads and find for yourself what you like. Holistic practices are just that, a practice, and to practice something you must first experiment. Please give these suggestions a try, experiment, find what you like, and create an individual holistic practice that suits you and your family. The suggestions in the book are guidelines to help you get started. As you continue on you may create your own recipes and come up with other ideas you love and are good for you.

Eating healthy need not be difficult or take a long time. Some things are easy and quick and still very good for you. You just have to train yourself to make those healthy choices and learn to create food in a healthy way. That is where these basics come in.

Soups: can be elaborate or very simple. The simplest way to make soup is to chop up various veggies, put in a pot, add enough broth to cover and cook until the veggies are done. When you poke a fork into them and they slide right off, that is when done. Depending on the size of the pot it will take as little as thirty minutes of cooking time, up to a couple of hours. Just put the stove on low and let it simmer until done.

Don't cook all soups either. If you want an even easier way to have soup, you can do raw soups. A raw soup is basically one you need not cook. You add all the ingredients to a blender, blend until smooth, and serve. There are a couple of recipes like that you may try. For those of you who may not feel up to trying to cook a soup, you can still have a healthy soup by making raw ones using fresh fruits and veggies and blending.

Stews: May take a little more work, but it is still an easy one pot meal for those on the go. Especially if you have a slow cooker at home, you can put everything into the slow cooker in the morning and when you get home you have a wonderful meal waiting for you ready to eat. You can do more than just stews in the slow cooker as you will find when you go through the recipes. I have a few great slow cooker recipes which are some of my favorite things to eat and are good for you too.

Veggie Dishes: Similar to salads, but using chopped veggies, adding them together and eating them either raw or slightly cooked. Very good and is quick and easy. Choose any variation of veggies you like, slice them up into similar sized pieces, put into a pan over medium heat and saute until heated. Don't make them over cooked, lightly sauteing veggies is good for you and helps to keep many nutrients intact, whereas overcooking can eliminate them.

Another great and tasty way to prepare and eat veggies is in roasting them. It may sound elaborate to some, but it's actually very simple. Just cut up various veggies, the best ones for roasting are root veggies like rutabaga, potatoes, carrots, onions, garlic, celery root, beets, and broccoli, cauliflower, Brussels sprouts, parsnips, asparagus, peppers, and shallots. Toss them in olive oil with salt and pepper and any herbs or spices you might like, but it's unnecessary and spread on a cookie sheet covered in parchment paper, and roast at 400 degrees for about 30 minutes. Flip them at the 15-minute mark for best results.

This is just an introduction to the simplest and most basic meals, to help those of you who want to experiment and try out the simple things first. If you are new to cooking and preparing food this is a great way to start. And if you are a veteran cook, you can still use these guidelines to make a quick and easy meal when strapped for time, and go on to all the amazing recipes in the book and create for yourself something great for you and your family when you have more time.

As for those of you still learning, look at all the recipes, discover which ones sound good or seem easier than others and try them to start out. Allow yourself to learn and experiment so you can cook and eat well. In another chapter get your children involved if you have any, this is a great way to instill healthy eating and make it fun. Let them learn how to cook as you learn how to eat holistically. Make it a family practice, they will thank you later. Some of my fondest memories involve cooking in the kitchen with my mom, learning how to bake, and having fun. Do that for you and your family. If you have no family yet, allow yourself to practice these things until they become a habit so that if you have a family you will have these skills to pass on to them and their children.

Cooking and family connections around preparing meals is often lost now, but is an important thing to bring back. It creates confidence, healthy choices, connections, and bonding. Which will take everyone further in life as they get older. This is an investment in you, your family, and future generations. Please make the most of it by feeding yourself and your family the best foods you can to ensure long life, health, and happiness. Because when you feel good inside you will feel good outside.

Chapter 10

The Tools of the Trade

There are tools that you have in your kitchen that you will need to cook and eat holistically. I made a list of things here to help you get it all together if you don't yet have some of it. Many things mentioned will be needed to make most recipes in the book as I make them. Here it goes:

Cast Iron
You will want a cast iron skillet for sure, and a dutch oven as well for bigger things like doing roasts and stews. Cast iron is the best tool to use for any cooking. It heats and cooks evenly, and it also adds extra iron to your meals, and this is great if you may be low or deficient in iron. It also cannot be destroyed. You can set it on fire and it won't hurt it. You may have to re-season it, but it will be okay. I use mine on the wood stove a lot, but I also use it on the regular cook stove and in the oven. That is part of what makes it so great is how versatile it is. Also easy to clean, you just rinse it with hot water, scrub with a sponge if needed, and NEVER use soap on it. Put it back on the stove, wipe it out with a towel to dry it, spray it with organic non-stick olive oil spray, and it's ready to go for next time.

Various Blenders
I have a basic Oster blender, a Ninja high powered blender, and a coffee grinder. You want the basic blender for everyday smoothies and the basics, a high powered blender for soups and bigger meals, then a coffee grinder or a small blender with a grinder attachment for making almond flour and oat flour. You can buy almond meal flour and oat flour at the store, but it's

good when you can make it on the spot at home. The choice is yours. I am just suggesting things for helping you get along holistically eating.

Food Processor

You will want this for making many things. You can also use this to make almond and oat flour, however, it may not grind it up as well and a coffee grinder will. The recipes that use this tool mentions food processor in them.

Stainless Steel

This is the best for stock pots. For making soups, stews, and much more. I love stainless steel, it is the second best material for cooking in next to cast iron. You don't want to use the nonstick pans, the coating on them leaves toxic chemicals in your food. That is why I only recommend either cast iron or stainless steel and nothing else. I know there are copper pans out there that many cooks recommend, however I have never used them and it is possible to get too much copper in your system and that would be bad. So I stick to my two choices. Do your research if you wish and discover which one would fit you best. Use your best judgment.

Juicer

With this, I am not talking about a high powered blender that some people call a juicer. What I am talking about is an actual juicer, a machine that turns fruits and vegetables into juice. I use a Jack Lalanne power juicer. There are many others out on the market, so look into it, do your research and get what you feel is best for you. This is a valuable tool to have in a healing kitchen.

Food Dehydrator

This is great for making apple chips and banana chips, as well as granola and re-drying soaked nuts and seeds. Can be used for so many healthy things so this is a great addition to your kitchen.

Recipes

Breakfast

Morning Smoothie

Italian Frittata

Basic Bran Muffins

Best Bran Muffins Ever

Greens and Eggs

Oatmeal Cookie Granola

Grain Free Granola

Breakfast Bars

Buckwheat Pancakes

Omelets

Easy No Cooking Breakfasts

Morning Smoothie
(Vegan)

What you will need:
Various fruits and vegetables of your choice
Try to make it be more vegetables than fruit.

Here is my usual:
One carrot
One celery stalk
One half zucchini
One half cucumber
One whole lemon or lime peeled

Juice all the ingredients listed above and put the juice in a blender.

Add in more fruits and vegetables easy to blend such as:
Sliced cored pear
One handful of kale or spinach
One cup of mixed berries (fresh or frozen)
One half to one whole avocado (depending on size)
Pineapple or mangoes

Blend in blender until smooth and enjoy.

Don't limit yourself to what I have mentioned here.
Eat the fruit and vegetables you like if they aren't listed here.
But also be willing to try new things too.
Experiment and enjoy the trial and error that comes with it.
Just use more vegetables than fruit and your good to go.

Italian Frittata

What you will need:

Preheat oven to 400 degrees.

Diced uncured nitrate free organic beef salami
Chopped artichoke hearts
Chopped sun-dried tomatoes
Fresh Spinach
6 Eggs (free range or organic)
1/3 cup plain unsweetened almond milk
Chopped onion
Chopped garlic
Fresh basil
Italian Seasoning Mix
Salt
Pepper
Organic Parmesan Cheese or Raw Goat Cheese (optional)

Now I don't have measurements or exact amounts of the meat and veggies because I feel it is personal how much or how little you like. This is how I cook, therefore this is how many of my recipes are. So gauge for yourself how much looks good, my rule of thumb is to have enough of the meat and veggies that it covers the bottom of the skillet. Also, make sure you have an oven proof skillet like cast iron since this will go in the oven.

Once you chop and dice the meat and veggies, cook them up in an ovenproof skillet over medium heat in olive oil.

Whisk the eggs, almond milk, seasonings, salt, and pepper in a bowl and pour over the meat and veggies in the skillet.

Bake for 20 minutes.
Pull it out of the oven and sprinkle the cheese on top if using.

Basic Bran Muffins

What you will need:

Preheat oven to 400 degrees.
Grease a 12 count muffin tin and set aside.

1/3 Cup organic butter or ghee
1/2 Cup coconut sugar
1 Egg (free range or organic)
1 tsp. Cinnamon
1 Cup Almond Meal Flour
1 tsp. Baking Powder
1/2 tsp. Baking Soda
1 tsp. Salt
1 Cup Almond Milk
3 Cups of Oat Bran

Cream butter, sugar, the egg, and cinnamon.
Add the flour, baking powder, baking soda, and salt until combined.
Then add the almond milk and oat bran alternately until well combined.
Put heaping spoonfuls of the batter into prepared muffin tin.
Bake for 20-25 minutes.

Best Bran Muffins Ever!

What you will need:

Preheat oven to 400 degrees.
Grease a 12 count muffin tin and set aside.

¾ cup Almond Meal Flour
¾ cup Oat bran
½ cup Coconut sugar
1 tsp. Baking powder
1 tsp. Cinnamon
½ Baking soda
1 mashed banana
½ cup plain unsweetened coconut yogurt
1 Egg (free range or organic)
2 Tbsp. Coconut Oil melted
½ tsp. Vanilla extract
1 small to medium carrot shredded
½ cup chopped dates
½ cup chopped walnuts (soaked for 4 hours)

Mix dry ingredients into a bowl first and set aside.
Next mix wet ingredients into a different bowl that's a little larger.
Add the dry ingredients to the wet ingredients and mix until just combined.
Fold in shredded carrot, dates, and walnuts.
Spoon into prepared muffin tin.
Bake for 18-20 minutes.

Greens and Eggs

What you will need:

Various organic greens such as:

Baby Kale
Spinach
Chopped Green Onions
Fresh Basil
Arugula

Two Eggs (free range or organic) Scrambled in a bowl with salt and pepper. You may add other dried herbs and spices if you like.

Heat a greased skillet with a tablespoon of coconut oil.
Put any the greens in the skillet and cook until slightly wilted.
Then add the eggs and let cook for a bit, then flip.
Cook until the desired doneness is achieved.
I don't like runny eggs, but some people do, so please cook them to your desired outcome.

Oatmeal Cookie Granola

(Vegan)

What you will need:

1 cup gluten-free oats
¼ cup flax seeds
3 Tbsp. Raw pumpkin seeds soaked overnight
6 Tbsp. Almond butter melted
3 Tbsp. Orange Date syrup (recipe below)
½ tsp. Vanilla extract
3 Tbsp. Dried cranberries
A pinch of Himalayan Pink Salt
The zest of one organic orange
1 tsp. Cinnamon

Combine all ingredients in a bowl, then press into an 8x8 glass dish and refrigerate for at least an hour before eating. Store in fridge.

Orange Date Syrup
1 orange juiced
1 cup chopped dates
Blended in a blender until a smooth paste forms.
Store in a jar in the fridge for up to a week.

Grain Free Granola
(Vegan)

What you will need:

¼ cup macadamia nuts soaked for an hour
3 Tbsp. Buckwheat groats soaked for 15 minutes
¼ cup almonds soaked overnight
½ tsp. Cinnamon
¼ tsp. Powdered ginger root
1 tsp. Vanilla extract
1/3 cup unsweetened coconut flakes
1 Tbsp. Coconut oil
2 Tbsp. Coconut milk
1 Tbsp. Raw Organic Honey or stevia (to make it vegan)

Put all ingredients into a food processor and process until chunky, but don't over process.
Put granola into a food dehydrator and dry for 6-8 hours at 95 degrees.

Notes: The reasoning behind soaking the groats and nuts prior to using them is to make them easier for the body to digest and use the nutrients contained.
Also, you want to keep the food dehydrator at 95 degrees or lower to keep the integrity of the raw honey intact since raw honey contains many healing properties you want to keep available. If raw honey is heated over that temperature then the nutrients will get depleted and that will defeat the purpose of using it.

Grain Free Breakfast Bars

(Vegan)

What you will need:

Preheat oven to 350 degrees.

¼ cup buckwheat groats soaked for 15 minutes
½ cup walnuts soaked for 4 hours
½ cup almonds soaked overnight
¼ flax meal (ground flax seeds)
2 Tbsp. Hemp seeds
2 Tbsp. Coconut oil
2 Tbsp. Unsweetened coconut yogurt
½ tsp. Liquid Stevia
1 tsp. Cinnamon

Combine all ingredients in a food processor and blend until chunky and sticky.
Form spoonfuls of the mix into bars on a cookie sheet covered with parchment paper.
Bake for 8 minutes on one side, then flip over and bake for another 8 minutes.
Let cool on a wire cooling rack.

Icing
½ Tbsp. Melted coconut oil
2 Tbsp. Unsweetened coconut yogurt
1 tsp. Raw organic honey melted or stevia
1 tsp. Cinnamon

Combine all the icing ingredients together until well blended.
Drizzle the icing onto the bars once the bars are cool.
Store bars in the fridge for up to a week or eat within two days.

Buckwheat Pancakes

(Vegan)

Note: This recipe is for one pancake, therefore you can multiply it by however many pancakes you want to make for however many people you are making them for.

What you will need:

¼ cup buckwheat groats (soaked for 15 minutes)
2 Tbs. Oats

Put these first two ingredients into a food processor or coffee grinder until well blended.

Put that mixture into a bowl and add the rest of the ingredients.

½ Tbs. Arrowroot powder
½ tsp. Baking powder
1 tsp. Cinnamon
pinch of sea salt
½ tsp. Vanilla
½ cup almond milk

Mix well until it looks like regular pancake batter. Not too thick and not too runny. You can add more or less almond milk until the right consistency is attained.

Heat a cast iron frying pan over medium heat, spray pan with nonstick cooking spray and pour batter into hot pan. Cook on one side until bubbles form on the top and flip over. Cook another couple minutes and remove pancake.

Serve with pure organic maple syrup and grass-fed butter.

Omelets

What you will need:

Eggs (free range or organic)

How many eggs depends on how many omelets you are making and for how many people. I usually use two eggs per person.
Veggies:
Spinach, kale, zucchini, squash, mushrooms, onions, garlic, shallots, peppers, green onions, avocados, and more.
Pre-cooked Meat: (Optional)
Organic beef, chicken, bison, turkey, uncured nitrate free salami, and natural chicken or beef sausage.
Organic Cheese: (Optional)
Raw goat cheese
Salt, pepper, and any other dried herbs or spices you like best.

Whip up your eggs in a bowl with the salt, pepper, herbs, and spices if using. Then heat a greased skillet over medium heat. Add some coconut oil to the skillet until melted. Then pour your scrambled eggs into the hot skillet over the oil.
Then flip the eggs over after about five minutes. And cook that side for another five minutes.
Then fill your omelet on one side with your choice of veggies, meat, and cheese if using and flip the other side over it and cook for about a minute. Then you are ready to serve.

You can choose however many veggies you want from this list, you can even come up with your own if I have missed anything here. Again this is a great recipe to experiment with and try different variations. Also, you can use as much or as little meat or cheese you wish if it will fit in your omelet.

Easy No Cooking Breakfasts

Gluten Free Toast With Almond Butter
Udis is a good brand of gluten-free bread.
You can also try your hand at making your own gluten-free bread.
My favorite brand of almond butter is Barney Butter. It is so tasty, plus a bare smooth version doesn't have any added sugars or salt and it still tastes wonderful.

Gluten Free Toast With Smashed Berries
Get a handful of fresh berries and smash them into a piece of gluten-free toast, then eat.

Gluten Free Toast With Smashed Avocado.
Put the inside of the avocado in a bowl, stir and smash it till somewhat smooth and spread over the toast.

Granola With Almond or Coconut milk.
If you don't want to make your own granola you can always buy organic gluten free granola and eat it with your milk of choice for an easy no-cook breakfast.

Gluten Free Instant Oatmeal
I like the Glutenfreeda brand.
For those on the go who need it real quick.

Smoothies
I already have a smoothie recipe in the book, but I have to list it here as a reminder because it is a great no cooking breakfast you can take on the go if you need to.

Protein Shake
You can also get yourself a blender bottle and have protein shakes for breakfast. Just put some almond milk, or other milk of choice into the bottle, add a scoop of protein powder, shake and go.

All these breakfasts can be done alone or in combination. I often have a muffin, eggs, or granola, along with my morning smoothie. For myself, I have found that a smoothie alone doesn't fill me enough anymore, so I need to eat more than just that. These recipes and suggestions are good and healthy and are a great way to transition to a holistic way of eating. Start with breakfast, that's what I did. Change one thing by trying one recipe out as your breakfast for a week and see how you feel. I know many people these days don't even eat breakfast and it is important to do so. Your body needs the right fuel to function throughout the day and I am sorry to tell you that just coffee is not the proper way to fuel your body. It can actually be very harmful, especially if you aren't eating anything with it. Ditch the coffee if you can, if not, make sure it's organic and at least learn to eat a healthy breakfast with it, your body will thank you.

Once you do you will feel more energy because your body will be fueled in the way it was meant to be fueled and will function better overall because of that. It also helps your brain function better making you better able to tackle anything that comes your way, you will feel less frazzled and less stressed when your brain is fueled right. That is why it's good to switch to a holistic way of eating, to fuel your body right, to get the right amount and the right nutrients into your body, so you may function at full capacity in all ways and feel good doing it.

Main Dishes

(Can be used for lunch or dinner.)

Chicken with Spinach and Artichokes

Slow Cooker Chicken Chili

Basic Red Sauce

Chicken, Squash, Zucchini Saute

Basic Beef Stew

Mediterranean Rice Bowl

Veggie Taco Bake

Taco Salad

Chicken Stew

Beef Roast

Detox Rice

Veggie Chili

Southwest Chicken Casserole

Ground Meat and Veggies

Marinara Sauce

Chicken Marinara

Brussels Sprouts Rice Bowl

Easy No Cooking Main Dishes

Chicken with Spinach & Artichokes

What you will need:

Preheat oven to 400 degrees

Two Chicken Breasts (free range or organic)
1 cup baby spinach
1 small can artichokes chopped
½ onion chopped
2 carrots chopped
2 garlic cloves diced
1 cup chicken stock
olive oil
sea salt
pepper

Salt and pepper the chicken, brown it on both sides in a greased pan, then set aside.
Heat oil in cast iron or oven proof skillet.
Add all veggies except the spinach and cook until slightly tender
Then add the spinach, the browned chicken, and the chicken stock.
Put in the oven and bake for 20 minutes.

Additions: You can also add sun-dried tomatoes, sliced olives, kale, and sprinkle with goat cheese after pulling out of the oven. You can have it as simple as the main recipe, or as elaborate, by adding more to it, as you want.

Part of cooking is experimenting and trying new flavors and combinations. Have fun with it and see where you take it.
You might find something amazing that you love and want to cook again and again.

Slow Cooker Chicken Chili

What you will need:

½ onion chopped
1 can organic kidney beans
1 can organic black beans
1 can organic tomatoes
2 cups frozen organic corn
1 jar organic tomato sauce (I use Bertolli Organic Pasta Sauce)
Cumin
Chili powder
Garlic powder
Onion powder
Dried oregano
Paprika
Salt
Pepper
Two to Three Chicken Breasts (free range or organic)

Again I did not put measurements for the seasonings because I don't measure them out, this is personal preference. Use what you like and use how much you think you will like. It's kind of a form of intuitive eating, where you listen to your intuition regarding what you want to eat and how you want to eat it, well it can also work with how much or how little you want to season it. So go with what looks good to you. Just try not to overdo it.

Put all ingredients into a slow cooker and cook on low for about 6-8 hours depending on how hot your slow cooker cooks. Mine cooks on the hot side so it only takes about six hours, but yours may take longer. My rule of thumb is that if you stick a fork into the chicken and the chicken falls apart it is done and ready. Shred chicken in the pot after the cooking time is done and stir well. Serve with organic cheese, cilantro, chopped onions, and sliced black olives.

Basic Red Sauce
(Vegan)

One of the best things you can do is make your own pasta sauce, most of the store bought one contain added sugars and other unhealthful additives like preservatives you don't want in your body. You can buy organic pasta sauces, but making your own tastes wonderful and saves you money.

What you will need:

Olive oil
Chopped Garlic
Fresh Chopped Parsley and Basil
1 Can Pureed Tomatoes (or four fresh tomatoes pureed in a blender)
Salt
Pepper
Organic Butter or Ghee

There are no measurements yet again, I know some of you will really hate me for that, but like I said this is how I cook, so many of my recipes don't have measurements. For this recipe, it depends on how much you want to make, how many people you are feeding, or if it's only for yourself.

Using one can of tomatoes, or four fresh ones will yield enough for a double serving, meaning it will serve two people. Therefore if you are serving four people double it, and so forth.

Use as much garlic and herbs as you like, they are so good for you and taste wonderful. So experiment and see what you like. It's part of the fun of cooking.

Cook the garlic in the olive oil until soft, add the parsley and basil just until wilting, then add the tomatoes, salt and pepper to taste, and cook for about 15 minutes. Then add a spoonful of the butter or ghee, stir and serve. Best served with gluten-free pasta of choice, or even zucchini noodles. You can even sprinkle on some goat cheese to top it off.

Chicken, Squash, Zucchini Saute

This is one of the easiest meals you can make and it's good too.

What you will need:

2 Tbsp. Olive Oil
½ shallot diced
1 large chicken breast cubed (free range or organic)
1 medium crookneck squash chopped
1 medium zucchini chopped
Salt
Pepper

If you have a wok it works best with this recipe, however if not, you can use a skillet too.

Heat oil in a skillet, cook shallot until softened, add squash and zucchini and cook until they soften.
Add cubed chicken, salt, and pepper, and saute until the chicken is done.

Serve

Basic Beef Stew

Preheat oven to 350 degrees

What you will need:

1 Package of Grass Fed Beef Stew Meat
Many root vegetables cubed
      carrots
      potatoes
      parsnips
      rutabagas
      celery root
      beets
      turnips
1 onion chopped
2 garlic cloves diced
salt and pepper

You can use these roots together, or just choose a few you like.
How many you use will depend on the size of your skillet and how many people you are serving.
Heat oil in a cast iron dutch oven over medium heat
Cook the onion and garlic until softened
Brown the meat with some salt and pepper
Next, add all the vegetables you plan to use and cover with water or beef broth whichever one you have will work fine. Then put in the preheated oven for about an hour. Check it periodically, stirring occasionally, it will be done when the vegetables are done.

Serve with sauteed greens or a salad to round out the meal.

Mediterranean Rice Bowl

What you will need:

Olive oil
½ onion chopped
2 cloves garlic chopped
1 chicken breast cubed
1 small crookneck squash cubed
1 small zucchini cubed
1 small can artichoke hearts
1 can sliced olives
¼ cup sun-dried tomatoes
Fresh basil, oregano, and parsley (you can use dried if that's all you have)
Sea salt and black pepper
Organic Parmesan cheese (optional)
2 servings of Pre-cooked white basmati or jasmine rice

Heat oil in a skillet
Saute onion and garlic
Add chicken, sea salt, and black pepper.
Cook until browned on the outside.
Add the vegetables and cook until they are done.
Add the herbs until just wilted if using fresh.
Mix with the rice.
Serve with grated Parmesan cheese if using.

Veggie Taco Bake

Preheat oven to 350 degrees

What you will need:

Organic Tortilla Chips
Olive Oil
½ onion chopped
½ cup organic salsa (or homemade salsa)
2 garlic cloves diced
cumin
chili powder
1 small zucchini chopped
1 small crookneck squash chopped
1 can organic black beans
1 can organic yellow corn
½ cup organic chicken stock
1 can sliced black olives (optional, but good)
Pink Himalayan Salt
Black pepper
Organic cheese for topping (optional)

Heat oil in a skillet
Cook onion and garlic until softened
Add everything else except for cheese
Cook for about 5 minutes and turn off the heat.
Grease a 9x9 inch glass baking dish
Put a layer of the organic tortilla chips on the bottom of the baking dish
Pour the veggie mix over the chips
Add another layer of organic tortilla chips over the veggie mix
Top with organic cheese

Bake for 20-30 minutes until it bubbles.
If you have a clear glass pan you can see this.

Taco Salad

What you will need:

Olive oil
1 pound package of organic ground beef or bison
½ onion chopped
1 garlic clove diced
cumin
chili powder
paprika
sea salt
pepper
Sliced black olives
Organic Spring Mix or Other Organic Salad Greens
Organic Cheese
Organic or homemade salsa
Chopped Green Onions
Organic Tortilla Chips
Homemade Ranch Dressing (recipe page 89)

Heat oil in a skillet over medium heat
Add garlic and onion, cook, until softened.
Add ground meat and cook with the cumin, chili powder, paprika, salt, and pepper, until done.
Get out a nice big salad bowl, put your greens in it.
Load it up with the black olives, cheese, salsa, green onions, and crushed tortilla chips.

Chicken Stew

Preheat oven to 350 degrees

What you will need:

1-2 Chicken Breasts Cubed (Depends on how many you are serving)
1-2 carrots sliced
1-2 celery stalks chopped
1 large potato cubed
3 cloves of garlic cut in half
tarragon
salt
pepper
Chicken stock

Put everything in a cast iron skillet or dutch oven
Pour enough chicken stock in the pot to just cover everything
Put the cast iron in the oven and bake for 30 minutes

Beef Roast

Preheat oven to 350 degrees
What you will need:

Olive Oil
Grass Fed Beef Roast of Choice
Garlic
Onions
Water
Salt
Pepper

Heat oil in cast iron dutch oven.
Sprinkle the roast with salt and pepper on both sides
Brown the meat on all sides.
Chop garlic and onions and add to pot.
Fill with water until the roast is covered.
Place in oven and cook until meat falls apart.

I like to cook this on the wood stove, but since most people don't have that option the oven works great for this too. However, if you have a wood stove I would highly recommend trying this on it, it turns out so good. Do all the same things as mentioned above and cook it until it falls apart, you just do it on a wood stove instead of in the oven.

Serve with the sides in the book, or with a salad and enjoy.

Detox Rice

(Vegan)

What you will need:

1 tbsp. Olive oil
1 tbsp. Mustard seeds
1 tsp. Turmeric
1 tsp. Pink Himalayan Salt
1 tsp. Cumin
1 tsp. Powdered Ginger Root
1 tsp. Coriander
1 cup Basmati rice
1 Carrot chopped
1 Celery stalk chopped
2 cups Chicken Stock

Cook the spices in olive oil over medium heat for about 1 minute.
Add the Basmati rice and stir until combined.
Add in the vegetables and chicken stock, bring to boil.
Reduce heat to low.
Cook until the rice is done.
This could take up to 30 minutes and you may have to add more liquid as needed if it evaporates faster than the rice cooks. Keep an eye on it and stir it often to prevent sticking or burning.

Veggie Chili
(Vegan)

What you will need:

1 tbsp. Olive oil
1 tsp. Cumin
1 small onion chopped
2 cloves garlic diced
1 jalapeno diced with seeds removed
1 small zucchini chopped
1 small sweet potato chopped
1 can organic black beans
1 can organic kidney beans
1 can organic tomatoes
1 tsp. sea salt
chopped cilantro
handful of chopped kale
water

Heat olive oil in a stainless steel saucepan.
Add cumin, onion, and garlic.
Cook until softened.
Add the rest to the pot and fill with water until just covered.
Cook until the potatoes are done.
Serve with organic tortilla chips and guacamole.

Southwest Chicken Casserole

Preheat oven to 350 degrees

What you will need:

1 can organic black beans
1 can organic kidney beans
chopped green onions
sliced black olives
chopped roasted red pepper
½ cup of organic salsa
chopped pre-cooked chicken
salt
pepper
1 handful chopped fresh cilantro
Organic taco seasoning
1/2 red cabbage chopped
oregano
Shredded organic cheddar cheese for topping (optional)

Use your best judgment regarding the amounts of what you add to this dish depending on the number of people you are serving and how much you like certain ingredients. Make it fit your tastes.
Combine all ingredients in a bowl except for cheese.
Stir to combine well.
Transfer to a baking dish. Whatever size it will fit into is great.
Top with shredded cheese.
Bake for 15-20 minutes for an 8x8 in baking dish.
Bake for 25-30 minutes if making more and using a bigger baking dish.

Ground Meat & Veggies

What you will need:

1 tbs. olive oil
1 pound package of ground grass fed beef
1 package frozen peas and carrots combination
1 half onion chopped
salt and pepper

Heat oil in skillet over medium heat.
Cook chopped onion until softened.
Add meat and cook until almost done.
Add the veggies with salt and pepper.
Cover and cook until veggies are done.

Marinara Sauce

(Vegan)

What you will need:

½ cup olive oil
1 small onion chopped
1 large carrot chopped
1 can sliced black olives
2 garlic cloves diced
1 can organic diced tomatoes
1 jar organic pasta sauce (I like Bertoli's the best)
1 small can tomato paste
2 tbsp. Italian seasonings
1 tbsp. Honey (optional)
Salt and pepper

Heat oil in a skillet over medium heat.
Cook onion, carrots, and garlic until softened.
Add black olives and cook a few more minutes.
Transfer everything in the skillet to a slow cooker.
Add the diced tomatoes, pasta sauce, tomato paste, Italian seasonings, honey (if using,) salt and pepper. Stir well to combine.
Cook on low for about 5 hours.
Stirring occasionally.
Serve over gluten-free pasta noodles, zucchini noodles, or chicken.
Add a salad or other vegetable dish to round out the meal.

Chicken Marinara

Preheat oven to 350 degrees

What you will need:

Marinara sauce made ahead from the previous page.
However many chicken breasts you need per serving depending on how many people you are feeding. One chicken breast per person, or per couple depending on breast size.
Namaste Foods Gluten Free Bread Crumbs
Olive oil in a hot skillet
Organic Mozzarella cheese sliced (optional)

Put your chicken breasts in a bag with the bread crumbs and toss to combine.
Heat oil in a skillet over medium heat.
Put breaded chicken in the skillet and brown on both sides.
Then put the chicken breasts in a greased oven safe baking dish.
Once the chicken is breaded and browned in the baking dish cover with marinara sauce.
Put sliced mozzarella over the chicken, if using, then bake for 30 minutes.
Serve with a salad or other vegetables.

Brussels Sprouts Rice Bowl

Preheat oven to 400 degrees

What you will need:

2 cups chicken stock
½ cup white basmati rice
½ cup mixed wild rice
½ shallot diced
½ pound Brussels sprouts quartered
1 chicken breast precooked and shredded
olive oil
salt
pepper

Put chicken stock into a saucepan and bring to a boil. Add rice to boiling chicken stock. Cook rice over medium heat 25-30 minutes. Put in a bowl and set aside.

Put quartered Brussels sprouts, diced shallots, and shredded chicken into a baking dish, pour olive oil over it with salt and pepper. Toss to combine and bake for 30 minutes. Stirring at the halfway point.

Pull the baking dish out of the oven and add it to the bowl of rice. Toss to combine and serve.

Easy No Cooking Main Dishes

Raw soup (recipe to follow in the next chapter)

Salads:
with meat, nuts, seeds, and various vegetables to make it a full meal.
Refer to the salad page for further ideas.

Broccoli Slaw:
shredded broccoli tossed with salad dressing (homemade is best), nuts,
seeds, and fruit like chopped apples or dried cranberries.

Coleslaw:
Shredded cabbage and shredded carrots, tossed with salad dressing (again
homemade is best or organic if you don't want to make your own), nuts,
seeds, fruits, and you can even top it with meat if you want or serve it
alongside a meat dish.

These easy no cooking main dishes make great lunches, just make ahead
the night before and have them ready to take with you for lunch the next
day.

Soups

Bone Broth

Bone Broth Soup

Roasted Tomato Soup

Pumpkin Soup

Celery Root Soup

Detox Soup

Tortilla Soup

Tomato Black Bean Soup

Blended Veggie Soup

Roasted Zucchini Soup

Cabbage Soup

Rustic Butternut Squash Soup

Carrot Ginger Soup

Easy No Cooking Soups - Raw Tomato Soup

Bone Broth

What you will need:

Bones: beef femur bones, beef knuckle bones, or a whole chicken carcass.

Bones from grass-fed beef and free range chicken is best. Organic when possible.

If you buy a whole roasted chicken from the grocery store and eat most of the meat on it you can then use the leftover carcass, bones and all to boil out for bone broth and make soup with it.

One carrot cut in half
One onion quartered
One celery stalk cut in half
Two cloves of garlic cut in half

Put all ingredients into a slow cooker and cover with filtered water until the slow cooker is full, cook on low for 24 hours or more.

Store broth in glass jars in the fridge for up to a week, or freeze to keep for longer.

You can drink this like you would tea or coffee, warm bone broth on a cold day is a great way to stay warm and feeling good. You can also use this broth as a base for soups, to cook rice or vegetables in, and more. Any recipe that calls for broth or stock you can use this in its place.

Bone Broth Soup

What you will need:

Pre-made bone broth
Olive oil
Chopped vegetables: carrots, celery, onions, garlic, zucchini, kale.
Meat: Use chicken with chicken broth and beef with beef broth. Or don't use meat if you don't want to since the bone broth is full of protein and other nutrients that meat also contains.
Salt
Pepper
Italian Seasonings

Heat olive oil in a saucepan over medium heat.
Saute the vegetables until softened.
Add meat if using and cook until just browned on the outside.
Add salt, pepper, and Italian seasonings.
Cover with bone broth until well covered.
Cook over medium heat until boiling, then turn heat to low and simmer for about an hour.

Serve with a green salad or herb rice to round out the meal if needed.

Roasted Tomato Soup

What you will need:

Preheat oven 350 degrees

A half pound of fresh tomatoes or one can fire roasted tomatoes
½ onion sliced
1 garlic clove diced
1 cup broth (whatever kind of broth you want to use.)
1 cup of filtered water
1 tbs. Paprika
¼ tsp. Chili powder
1 cup plain almond milk

If using fresh tomatoes slice them and put into a baking dish
If using canned tomatoes open the can and put the contents into a baking dish liquid and all.
Put onions and garlic over the tomatoes.
Bake for one hour

Transfer to a blender add the remaining ingredients and blend until smooth. Then put into a saucepan and cook over medium heat until warm.

Serve with chips and avocados.

Pumpkin Soup

What you will need:

Olive oil
½ onion chopped
1 roasted red pepper sliced (you can find these canned in the condiment section of the grocery store usually with the olives and pickles.)
1 sweet potato cubed
1 garlic clove diced
1 tbs. Oregano
2 cups chicken broth
1 can organic pumpkin
salt
pepper

Heat oil in saucepan over medium heat.
Cook onion and garlic until softened.
Add oregano and stir to combine.
Add the rest of the ingredients and cook over medium heat until boiling.
Reduce heat to low and simmer until potatoes are done. When a fork poked into one comes out easily.

Put everything into a blender and blend until smooth.
Drizzle with balsamic vinegar to garnish. (optional)

Celery Root Soup

What you will need:

1 celery root peeled and chopped
1 carrot chopped
1 celery stalk chopped
½ onion chopped
1-inch chunk ginger root grated
Chicken Broth – enough to cover the vegetables
salt
pepper

Put all ingredients into a saucepan and cover with broth.
Add salt and pepper, stir to combine.
Cook over medium heat until boiling.
Reduce heat to low and simmer for one hour.

Put into a blender and blend until smooth.
Serve.

Don't blend it if you don't want to, I just like blended soups and most recipes that call for blending are unnecessary.
So really it's up to you if you want to blend them or not. As long as they are cooked you can eat them either way.

Detox Soup

What you will need:

Olive oil
½ onion chopped
2 cloves garlic diced
Chicken broth
chopped vegetables: potatoes, carrots, celery, zucchini
1 can tomatoes
1-inch chunk ginger root grated
2 tbs. Hot sauce
1 tsp. Red pepper flakes
1 tsp. Black pepper
1 tsp. Curry powder
1 tsp. Chili powder
1 tsp. Pink Himalayan salt
1 cup plain coconut milk

Heat oil in saucepan over medium heat.
Saute onions and garlic until softened.
Add chopped vegetables and saute them too.
Add broth and spices and heat to a boil.
Reduce heat to low and simmer for 30 minutes.
Remove from heat and add coconut milk.
Stir to combine and serve.

I recommend serving this with the Mint Tulip drink in the drink section. This soup is very spicy and hot and the mint drink helps cool the heat making it a great combination for detoxification and digestion.

The ginger and other spices in this soup help get the circulation moving which aids in detoxification and elimination. The mint in the Mint Tulip drink aids digestion and soothes the stomach lining. Ginger is also good for digestion. This soup/drink combination is good for the changing of the seasons as a mild cleanser for the internal system.

Tortilla Soup

What you will need:

Olive oil
5 cups chicken broth
1 and a half pounds of chicken breast cubed
1 onion chopped
1 garlic clove diced
1 small red pepper seeded and diced
1 medium zucchini chopped
1 tsp. Chili powder
1 tsp. Cumin
1 tsp. Oregano
salt
pepper
1 cup fresh or frozen organic corn kernels
1 can organic black beans
1 cup organic salsa (I love Costo's Kirkland Brand)
1/3 cup chopped fresh cilantro

Heat olive oil in saucepan over medium heat.
Saute garlic and onions until softened.
Add broth, chicken, red pepper, zucchini and spices.
Cover and cook about 10 minutes or until zucchini is softened.
Reduce heat to low, add the rest of the ingredients and simmer covered for 30 minutes, stirring occasionally.

Serve with organic tortilla chips, grated organic cheese, chopped green onions, and sliced black olives.

Tomato Black Bean Soup

What you will need:

Olive oil
1 onion chopped
1 clove garlic diced
1 can black beans
1 can fire roasted tomatoes
½ can black olives sliced
1 can organic corn
1 cup chicken broth
salt
pepper
paprika
cumin
chili powder

Heat olive oil over medium heat.
Saute onion and garlic until softened
Add the rest of the ingredients.
Use as much or as little of the spices as you like, if you want it less spicy use just a tiny bit, and if you want it more spicy use a little bit more. You can make these things to your tastes.
Heat until boiling, reduce heat to low.
Simmer for 30 minutes.
Serve.

Blended Veggie Soup

What you will need:

A big variety of vegetables.
Use whatever you would like or whatever you have on hand.
You can use any vegetables you want truly.
This will turn out great no matter what you choose.

Chop all the veggies and put into a saucepan.
Fill the pot with a broth of choice. Either vegetable broth, chicken broth, or bone broth.
Add salt, pepper, basil, oregano, and any other herbs you like.

Cook over medium heat until boiling.
Reduce heat to low and simmer for an hour.

Pour everything into a blender and blend until smooth.
Serve alone or with a meal.

Roasted Zucchini Soup

What you will need:

Preheat oven to 400 degrees

2 zucchinis sliced
½ onion sliced
½ shallot sliced
Olive oil
Salt
Pepper
Herbs of choice
Chicken Broth

Put zucchini, onion, and shallots on a baking sheet covered with parchment paper.
Drizzle with olive oil.
Sprinkle with salt, pepper, and whatever herbs you like.
I use Italian seasonings most often.

Roast in at 400 degrees for 15 minutes, then flip them over, and roast for another 15 minutes.
Take out of the oven and put into a blender, add enough broth to cover.
Blend until smooth, add more broth if needed so it's not too thick, but don't add too much or it will be too runny.
Put into a saucepan and heat until warm and serve.

Cabbage Soup

What you will need:

Olive oil
½ onion chopped
2 cloves garlic diced
2 carrots chopped
1 celery stalk chopped
½ cup diced uncured beef salami
½ green cabbage chopped and shredded
5 cups chicken broth
1 can white beans
1 sweet potato chopped
salt
pepper
Just a sprinkle of each herb:
basil
thyme
fennel
savory
marjoram
rosemary
sage

Heat oil in saucepan over medium heat.
Saute onions and garlic until softened.
Add carrots and celery and saute more.
Then add the rest of the ingredients and heat to boiling.
Reduce heat to low, simmer for 15-20 minutes until potatoes are done.

Rustic Butternut Squash Soup

What you will need:

Preheat oven to 375 degrees

Olive oil
1 Butternut Squash Roasted (directions below)
½ chopped onion
1 carrot chopped
1 celery stalk chopped
½ shallot chopped
2 garlic cloves diced
4 cups chicken broth
salt
pepper

Cut butternut squash in half lengthwise.
Lay on a cookie sheet and drizzle with olive oil
Put in oven and bake for 30 minutes.

Pull out of the oven and set aside.

Heat more olive oil in a saucepan over medium heat.
Saute onion, garlic, and shallots.
Add carrot and celery.
Scoop out the inside of the butternut squash and add that to the pot.
Discard the outer shell.
Add the rest of the ingredients and heat to boiling.
Reduce heat to low and simmer for 30 minutes, or until carrot is tender.

Put into a blender and blend until smooth.

Carrot Ginger Soup

(Vegan)

What you will need:

5 cups vegetable stock
1 pound of carrots chopped
2 teaspoons freshly grated ginger root
1 orange freshly juiced
salt
Pepper

Bring stock, carrots, and ginger to a boil over medium heat in a saucepan.
Reduce heat to low, simmering for about 45 minutes.
Or until carrots are very tender.
Remove from heat and put into a blender.
Blend with fresh orange juice, salt, and pepper.
Chill for four hours or overnight.
Serve cold.

This is served chilled.

Easy No Cooking Soup

Raw Tomato Soup
(Vegan)

What you will need:

1 can organic tomatoes or four fresh tomatoes sliced
1 roasted red pepper (you can buy this in a jar)
¼ cup sun-dried tomatoes (in a jar packed with olive oil)
¼ cup fresh cilantro chopped
2 celery stalks chopped
¾ cup of filtered water
The juice of half a lime
2 tbs. Olive oil
salt
cumin
chili powder
paprika

Add all ingredients to a blender and blend.
Serve with organic tortilla chips, sliced avocados, green onions, black olives, and organic cheese.

Side Dishes
& Dressings

Salads

Salad Dressings:
     Basic Salad Dressing
     Vinaigrette Dressing
     Goats Milk Kefir Ranch Dressing
     Gut Healing Avocado Dressing

Zucchini Carrot Patties

Shallot Brussels Sprouts

Sauteed Greens

Herb Rice

Roasted veggies

Guacamole

Sauteed Green Beans

Rutabaga Fries

Warm Carrot Broccoli Slaw

Oven Roasted Garlic Cabbage

Easy no cooking sides

Salads

Salads make a great side dish and they are quick and easy to put together. Since I already went over salads earlier in the book and you really can make them any way you like, I will just share with you some of my favorite homemade salad dressing recipes to top your salads with. Going with homemade is much better not only for taste, but because you know what is in it, they are natural, and have no additives which are what we are wanting to get away from. That makes these recipes great. Try them, adjust them to your tastes, and make them your own. These dressings will keep for up to a week in a tightly closed glass jar stored in the fridge.

Salad Dressings

Basic Salad Dressing (Vegan)
½ cup olive oil
juice of half a lemon
salt and pepper
herbs of choice
Put all ingredients into a small glass jar, shake, and serve.

Vinaigrette Dressing
1 Tbs. Organic Dijon Mustard
1/3 cup Sherry Vinegar
½ small shallot diced
pinch coarse salt
2/3 cup olive oil
1 tsp. Raw organic honey
pinch coarse black pepper
Put all ingredients into a small glass jar, shake, and serve.

Goat's Milk Kefir Ranch Dressing

2 tbsp. Plain goats milk yogurt or plain unsweetened coconut yogurt
½ cup Plain Goat's milk kefir
1 tbsp. Pre-made ranch dressing seasoning mix (directions below)

Combine the yogurt, kefir, and seasoning mix in a jar, shake, and serve.

Ranch Dressing Seasoning Mix
(make ahead of time and keep on hand)
2 tbsp. Dried basil
2tbsp. Dried parsley
1 tbsp. Onion powder
1 tbsp. Garlic powder
1 tbsp. Dried oregano
1 tsp. Pepper.
Combine these dried ingredients together in a small jar to keep in the pantry for making dressings with. Give it a good shake before using.

Gut Healing Avocado Dressing

½ cup Plain goat's milk kefir
1 Tbs. Plain goat's milk yogurt
1 ripe avocado (peel and seed removed)
salt and pepper

Put all ingredients into a blender or food processor and blend until well combined. Store in a small glass jar.

Zucchini Carrot Patties

What you will need:

2 medium zucchinis shredded
1 small carrot shredded
2 green onions diced
2 cloves of garlic diced
1 egg
½ cup gluten-free flour
½ tsp. Baking powder
pinch of salt

Take shredded zucchini and carrots and put into a collider and let sit for a few minutes to drain.
Then add all ingredients into a dry and clean mixing bowl and mix well.
Heat a tablespoon of olive oil over medium heat in a cast iron skillet.
Scoop the batter into the hot skillet at the desired size.
Cook for about five minutes and flip, then cook another five minutes.
Serve.

Shallot Brussels Sprouts

(Vegan)

What you will need:

olive oil
½ pound Brussels Sprouts cleaned and quartered
1 shallot diced
1 tsp. Sherry vinegar
salt
pepper
herbs of choice
1 tbs. organic butter or ghee (optional)

Heat oil in a skillet over medium heat.
Add diced shallots and cook until lightly browned.
Add the cleaned and quartered Brussels Sprouts with salt and pepper
Cook until lightly browned.
Add the rest of the ingredients (except butter or ghee) and simmer for 5-10 minutes depending on the size of the Brussels Sprouts.
Remove from heat and add the tablespoon of butter or ghee if using, and serve.

Sauteed Greens

What you will need:

Olive oil
Chopped onion or shallot
Fresh Greens of choice
I use cabbage, green onions, kale, arugula, and spinach
Salt
Pepper
Herbs of choice
Splash of chicken broth
1 Tbs. Butter or ghee

Heat oil in a skillet over medium heat.
Add onion or shallot and cook until lightly browned.
Add in handfuls of greens and cover with lid.
Stir greens as they wilt and add the rest of the ingredients.
Cover and cook for about five minutes.
Stir more and add more greens if you feel it's necessary. Once sauteed greens get small so you can get away with using much more than you would if they were raw.
Cook until all greens are wilted and soft.
Add butter at the end and stir until well melted and combined.
Serve.

Herb Rice

What you will need:

Olive oil
½ onion chopped
½ cup white rice (Basmati and Jasmine are best)
1 ½ cups chicken stock or broth
salt
pepper
Fresh herbs diced (basil, oregano, parsley,)
Or if you don't have fresh you can use a dried Italian Seasoning Mix

Heat oil in a skillet over medium heat.
Saute chopped onion until softened.
Add rice and stir until combined.
Add the rest of the ingredients and reduce heat to low. Cook for 20-30 minutes until rice is done.
Serve.

Roasted Veggies

Preheat oven to 400 degrees

What you will need:

Olive oil
Vegetables for roasting
      potatoes
      carrots
      sweet potatoes
      rutabagas
      parsnips
      turnips
      onion
      garlic
      beets
      broccoli
Salt and pepper

You can use any combination of these vegetables or all of them.
Clean and chop them all to be around the same size pieces.
If you use garlic you want to use the whole clove and keep the skins on or they will burn. You will remove the skins after they are cooked.
If you use broccoli you will want to add it in the last 15 minutes of cooking or they too will burn.
The rest can all be cooked together for the same time.

Combine all clean chopped vegetables into a large mixing bowl.
Add enough olive oil to coat them all.
Add salt and pepper.
Toss to combine everything.
Put a piece of parchment paper over a cookie sheet and spread vegetables evenly over the sheet. Put in preheated oven and bake for 15 minutes.
Then stir and flip (add broccoli if using) and bake for another 15 minutes.

Guacamole

What you will need:

2 ripe avocados peal and seed removed
½ cup plain kefir (or plain yogurt if kefir isn't available)
1 cup of organic salsa
juice of half a lime

Put all ingredients into a blender and blend well.
Pour into a bowl and serve.

This is my quick and easy guacamole recipe. I know there are other ways to do it, but I like this best. For those of you who have never made your own, this is a great and easy way to start.

Serve with chips, sliced veggies, beans and rice, and more.

Sauteed Green Beans

What you will need:

Olive oil
Chopped onion or shallot
1 pound of fresh green beans cleaned and cut
Salt
Pepper
Splash of chicken broth

Heat olive oil in a skillet over medium heat.
Add onion or shallot and cook until lightly browned.
Then add the rest of the ingredients, cover, and cook stirring occasionally until green beans are done.
Serve.

Rutabaga Fries

Preheat oven to 400 degrees

What you will need:

One to two rutabagas depending on size and how much you want to make
Olive oil
Salt
Pepper
Paprika
Cumin
Onion Powder

Peel and slice rutabagas into fry-sized pieces about the same size as best as you can.
Toss into a bowl with the seasoning and coat.
Put parchment paper on a cookie sheet and spread the fries onto the sheet evenly.
Bake for 15 minutes.
Flip
Bake for another 15 minutes.
Serve with homemade ranch dressing.

Warm Carrot Broccoli Slaw

What you will need:

olive oil
2 cups shredded broccoli
2 cups shredded carrots
2 cloves garlic diced
salt and pepper

Heat oil in a skillet over medium heat.
Cook garlic until golden brown.
Add the rest of the ingredients and cook until softened.
Serve.

Oven Roasted Garlic Cabbage

Preheat oven to 400 degrees

What you will need:

1 green cabbage cut into round slices
3 Tbs. Olive oil
5 cloves of garlic diced
sea salt
pepper

Put sliced cabbage onto a baking sheet with parchment paper on it.
Cover the cabbage with the oil.
Spread diced garlic evenly over the cabbage.
Salt and pepper them.
Bake for 20 minutes, then flip over and bake for another 20 minutes.
Serve.

Easy No Cooking Sides

Chopped Veggies – Any vegetables of choice chopped and served with the main dish makes an easy go-to side dish.

Salads – Salad greens in a bowl with salad dressing is another quick and easy thing to add to the main dish as a side.

Shredded Carrots and Zucchini – Just shred a carrot with a small zucchini and toss with salt and pepper or serve with salad dressing over it.

Broccoli slaw – Shred broccoli and serve with salt and pepper or dressing.

Black bean and corn salad – Toss precooked and cooled black beans with organic corn, salsa, salt, and pepper, and serve with guacamole. This could also be eaten as a main dish on its own since it makes up a complete protein with the black bean corn combination.

Side Note: Black beans and rice together also make a complete protein for future reference if you are trying to get away from eating meat, you want to make sure you are consuming complete proteins and that is where proper food combinations come in.

Drinks

Fruity Water

Rainbow's Hot Day Cooler

Ginger Tea

Mineral Broth

Mint Tulip

Strawberry Lemonade

Strawberry Mango Cooler

Healthy Shamrock Shake

Orange, Carrot, Pineapple Juice

Detox Tea

Cacao Protein Shake

Oatmeal Cookie Shake

Hot Apple Cider

Dairy Free Hot Cocoa

Coconut Limeade

Raspberry Lime Water

Strawberry Kiwi Mojito Mock-tail

Fruity Water

What you will need:

A one-gallon glass jug or jar
Filtered water to fill jug or jar

Assorted fruits
Sliced:
strawberries
lemons
limes
oranges
cucumber
pineapple

Whole:
blueberries
raspberries
mint leafs

Put whatever fruits you choose into the jug or jar.
Fill with filtered water.
Keep in the fridge and drink daily.
Allow some of the fruit to end up in your glass and eat it.

Some nutrients from the fruit goes into the water so this makes it nutritional water. It also tastes good which is helpful for those who aren't big water drinkers get started on drinking water regularly. Plus it's pretty and looks like a cocktail without all the "bad" stuff.

Rainbow's Hot Day Cooler

What you will need:

A juicer

1 lemon juiced
1 apple juiced

Put the lemon and apple juice into a blender and add:
Fresh or frozen strawberries
Fresh or frozen mixed berries
Fresh or frozen pineapple
Crushed ice
1 Tbs. Agave or raw organic honey

Blend in blender until berries are well blended.
Serve.

My nickname as a kid was Rainbow and I came up with this original recipe in high school. I have since adapted it to be a more health-conscious version that still tastes great. Enjoy!

Ginger Tea

What you will need:

2 quart sauce pan filled with filtered water
1 Inch chunk of ginger grated
juice of half a lemon
1 tsp. Vanilla extract
1 tsp. Cinnamon

Put all ingredients into the sauce pan with filtered water.
Heat over medium heat and simmer for about 30-40 minutes.
Remove from heat and serve hot or allow it to cool and serve cold.

You can also sweeten this if you like with either agave, pure maple syrup, or raw organic honey, once it has cooled.

Store in the fridge for up to a week.
Drink daily.
This is a great tea for the digestive and detoxification systems.

Mineral Broth

What you will need:

2 large carrots
3 potatoes
1 cup kale
2 large celery stalks
1 onion
½ cup parsley
2 liters of filtered water
Pinch of sea salt

Heat in large stock pot until boiling.
Reduce heat to low.
Simmer all ingredients for a couple of hours.
Drain the liquid into a large glass jar or pitcher.
That's your mineral broth.
You can also blend the leftover veggies in a blender and make a blended soup to eat.

Both things are great for detoxification and cleansing.
While also eating a clean vegetable-based diet.

Mint Tulip

What you will need:

One cup peppermint tea brewed ahead of time and cooled to room temperature.
½ cup plain goat's milk kefir or plain coconut yogurt.
6-8 fresh peppermint leaves rinsed.
1 tbs. Raw organic honey
crushed ice

Put all ingredients into a blender and blend until smooth.
Serve.

This is a great accompaniment for hot spicy dishes like my detox soup.
Any time I make that soup I make this up to go with it.
It's cooling where the soup is heating, and they compliment each other well for that reason.
This is also very good for the digestive system.

Strawberry Lemonade

What you will need:

A juicer

1 apple juiced
one lemon juiced

Put the apple and lemon juice in a blender
Add sliced fresh strawberries
Crushed ice
Blend until well combined

You can also add more sliced strawberries when you serve it to make it look pretty.

Strawberry Mango Cooler

What you will need:

1 cup plain coconut water or vanilla coconut milk
6 sliced strawberries
4 chunks mango
crushed ice (optional)

Blend in a blender until smooth and serve.

Healthy Shamrock Shake

What you will need:

1 cup sliced frozen banana
1 cup spinach leaves
1 cup vanilla almond milk
2 drops vanilla extract
2 drops peppermint extract
5 fresh peppermint leaves (optional)

Blend in a blender until smooth and serve.

Orange, Carrot, Pineapple Juice

What you will need:

A juicer

1 large orange
1 large carrot
A handful of pineapple chunks

Juice all ingredients and serve.

This is my favorite juice treat.
I rarely do it due to the sugar content, but it's so yummy.
It makes a nice drink for something special.

To do this as a smoothie: (if you don't have a juicer)
Orange slices
Sliced carrot
Frozen pineapple chunks
Vanilla Almond Milk

Blend all ingredients in a blender until smooth and serve.

Detox Tea

What you will need:

A sprinkle of all these spices
turmeric
coriander
cumin
fennel seeds
cinnamon

Sliced ginger
1-2 green tea bags
1 peppermint tea bag
lemon slices

1 quart Boiling water

Put all ingredients into a heatproof pitcher or glass jar.
Steep for 20-30 minutes.
Strain and serve.

Cacao Protein Shake

What you will need:

One cup of almond milk
One tablespoon cacao powder
One scoop of vanilla protein powder (I use MRM Veggie Protein)
One tablespoon of date syrup (I make my own. Recipe at the bottom.)
Sprinkle of cinnamon
Splash of pure vanilla extract

I put it all in a blender bottle, shake it up, and go.

You can also put it in a high powered blender and add more to it like nuts,
oats, bananas, and other such things if you choose.
Experiment and see what you like.

Date Syrup

What you need:

One orange freshly juiced
One small apple freshly juiced
One cup of chopped dates
Freshly squeezed lemon juice from half a lemon

Blend in blender until creamy and blended.
Put into a glass jar with a tight fitting lid and store in the fridge.

This recipe I shared on my blog because I loved it so much.

Oatmeal Cookie Shake

What you will need:

1 cup plain goat's milk kefir or plain coconut yogurt
2 tbs. Oat bran
2 tbs. Ground flax seeds
1 tsp. Cinnamon
1 tsp. Vanilla extract
4 prunes soaked in warm water

Put all ingredients into a blender and blend until smooth, then serve.

Hot Apple Cider

What you will need:

Large Stock Pot
I pound of organic apples of choice, peeled, cored, and sliced.
Filtered Water - enough to cover the apples
1 tsp. Cinnamon
1 tsp. Ginger
1 Package of organic mulling spices

Boil until apples are tender, add more water ass needed so you have enough to actually make cider or else you will end up with apple sauce instead. Which is fine, you can still eat it but it won't work as cider if there isn't enough liquid.

Strain cider from the apples into a large glass jug or giant bowl.
Serve warm.

Dairy Free Hot Cocoa

What you will need:

1 cup vanilla almond milk
1-2 Tbs. Cacao powder
1-2 Tbs. Agave or raw honey
Pinch of cinnamon

Heat vanilla almond milk in a small saucepan over medium heat until steaming. Add cacao powder and stir well. Remove from heat and add natural sweeteners listed above and a pinch of cinnamon if you choose. Serve hot.

Coconut Limeade

What you will need:

2 cups crushed ice
1 cup of coconut milk
2 limes juiced
1 Tbs. Agave or raw honey

Blend in blender and serve with lime wedges.

Raspberry Lime Water

What you will need:

6 oz. A container of raspberries rinsed
2 limes quartered
1 32 oz. A container of coconut water
Ice Cubes
2-quart jug with lid

Squeeze berries and put into the jug.
Squeeze each quarter of lime and put each into the jug.
Fill with coconut water. Secure lid and shake.
Then add ice cubes and serve.

Strawberry Kiwi Mojito

What you will need:

1 cup of frozen strawberries
1 cup peeled, sliced, frozen kiwi
8 fresh mint leaves
1 cup crushed ice
1 cup liquid of choice (almond milk, coconut milk, coconut water)

Blend in blender and serve.

This is a great drink for those social gatherings where others may be drinking or you just want to look like you have something fun to drink without the alcohol. I don't drink anymore as a choice for my health and wellness and this is a great alternative.

Desserts

To be consumed occasionally.
Best to be consumed only once a week or less for your best health.

Rhubarb Oat Crumble

Gluten Free Dairy Free Strawberry Shortcakes

Gluten Free Chocolate Chip Cookies

Gluten Free Shortbread Cookies

Raw Brownie Bites (Vegan)

Dairy Free Raw Fudge (Vegan)

Orange you glad you got cranberries and walnuts in your oatmeal cookies

Buckwheat Spice Cookies

Easy Deserts That Require Little to No Cooking

Rhubarb Oat Crumble

Preheat oven to 375 degrees

What you will need:

For the Crumble:
¾ cup gluten-free flour blend (Namaste Foods is great.)
½ cup gluten-free oats
½ cup of coconut sugar
½ cup chopped walnuts
pinch of sea salt
¼ cup of organic butter or coconut oil

For the Filling:
1 cup of coconut sugar
2 Tbs. Organic corn starch
3 pounds of chopped rhubarb
1 Tbs. Pure Vanilla

Mix crumble ingredients together in a large bowl until it clumps.
Put in freezer while you do the filling.
For the filling put the coconut sugar and cornstarch in a bowl and mix well. Toss the rhubarb and vanilla in the coconut sugar-cornstarch mixture until well coated.
Put the filling ingredients into a well-oiled glass baking dish.
Pull crumble topping out of the freezer and pour over the top of the filling.
Bake for 45 minutes or until topping is golden brown and the filling is bubbling.
Serve warm with organic vanilla ice cream or coconut ice cream.

Gluten Free, Dairy Free Strawberry Shortcakes

Preheat oven to 425 degrees

What you will need:

2 Cups Gluten Free Flour Blend
2/3 cup Almond Milk
1 egg
3 tsp. Baking Powder
1/3 Cup Coconut Sugar
½ tsp. Salt
8 TBS Butter

Sliced Strawberries
Pure Organic Maple Syrup

Combine all the shortcake ingredients until it resembles coarse crumbles. Using floured hands, bring the dough together in a ball and roll out onto a floured surface. Cut into biscuit sized circles.
Bake for 10 minutes and let cool.

Slice strawberries if you don't have pre-sliced ones.
Put in a bowl and drizzle with one to two tablespoons of pure organic maple syrup and let sit.

Once the shortcakes/biscuits are cool slice them in half and fill with the strawberries and maple syrup combination.

Serve.

Gluten Free Chocolate Chip Cookies

Preheat oven to 350 degrees

What you will need:

1 Stick of Butter at Room Temperature
¾ Cup Coconut Sugar
1 tsp. Vanilla
1 egg
1 Cup Gluten Free Baking Mix
½ tsp. Baking Soda
½ tsp. Baking Powder
½ tsp. Salt

3/4-1 Cup Dark Chocolate Chips (fair trade is best)
Parchment paper covered cookie sheet

Cream butter and sugar together until well combined.
Add egg and vanilla and beat until smooth.
Add the rest of the ingredients until a soft dough forms.
Then add in a 3/4-1 cup of Dark Chocolate Chips
Fold in until well distributed.

Cover and refrigerate for 1 hour.

Using a teaspoon spoon out balls of dough and put on a cookie sheet covered with parchment paper. Bake in the oven at 350 degrees for 8-10 minutes. Remove from oven and let cool for 5 minutes before removing from cookie sheet.

Gluten Free Shortbread Cookies

Preheat oven to 400 degrees

What you will need:

½ Cup Gluten Free Flour Blend
¼ Cup Coconut Sugar
¼ Cup Butter
¼ tsp. Salt
½ tsp. Vanilla extract

Combine all ingredients in a bowl until a soft dough forms.
Roll into balls and place on a cookie sheet covered with parchment paper.
Flatten balls with the backside of a fork that's been dipped in water.
Bake for 8-10 minutes.
Let sit for 5 minutes on cookie sheet before removing.

Raw Brownie Bites

(Vegan)

What you will need:

1 ½ Cups Walnuts
¼ Cup Cacao Powder
1 tsp. Vanilla
¼ tsp. Salt
1 Cup Prunes
1 TBS Water
1 TBS Pure Organic Maple Syrup

Combine all ingredients into a food processor and process until a dough-like a ball forms. Roll into balls using a tablespoon to spoon it out with. Roll the balls into cacao powder. Place on a plate or in a bowl and freeze for 15 minutes to set. Then keep refrigerated.

This is a great protein packed go-to snack.

Dairy Free Raw Fudge

(Vegan)

What you will need:

¾ Cup of Raw Cocoa Butter Melted
½ Cup Almond Butter
½ Cup Pure Organic Maple Syrup
1 TBS Coconut Oil
2 tsp. Vanilla
Pinch of Pink Himalayan Salt
½ Cup Chopped Nuts (Optional and you can use whatever nuts you like)

Combine all ingredients in a saucepan over a double boiler, or just over another saucepan with boiling water in it. Stir until well melted and combined. Spoon into candy/fudge molds.
Freeze for 1 Hour to set.
Store in the refrigerator.

Orange you glad you got cranberries and walnuts in your oatmeal cookies?

This is one of my all time favorite cookies. YUM!

Preheat oven to 375 degrees

What you will need:

1 Cup Gluten Free Flour Blend
1 tsp. Baking Powder
½ tsp. Cinnamon
¼ tsp. Nutmeg
½ Cup Butter
¾ Cup Coconut Sugar
1 egg
¼ Cup Almond Milk
1 tsp. Grated orange peel
1 ½ Cups Gluten Free Oats
¾ Cup Dried Cranberries
¼ Cup Chopped Walnuts

Combine all ingredients in a bowl until a soft dough forms.
Spoon out onto a parchment paper covered cookie sheet.
Bake for 9 minutes.
Remove from oven and let sit for 5 minutes before removing from cookie sheet.

Buckwheat Spice Cookies

Preheat oven to 350 degrees

What you will need:

1 Cup Buckwheat Flour
1 Cup Gluten Free Oats
¼ Cup Chopped Almonds
¼ Cup Coconut Sugar
½ tsp. Baking Soda
¼ tsp. Cream of Tar Tar
¾ tsp. Powdered Ginger
¾ tsp. Cinnamon
¼ tsp. Cardamom
¼ tsp. Salt
¼ Cup Melted Coconut Oil or Butter (Either works great.)
¼ Cup Pure Organic Maple Syrup
1 tsp. Vanilla
1 egg

Combine all ingredients and stir until a soft dough forms.
Spoon out and roll into balls.
Get a small plate and put some extra coconut sugar on it.
Roll balls into the plate of coconut sugar.
Place on a parchment paper covered cookie sheet.
Bake for 9 minutes.
Enjoy!

Easy Deserts That Require Little to No Cooking

Dairy-Free Ice Cream
Options: Coconut Ice Cream
Almond Milk Ice Cream
Cashew Milk Ice Cream

Goat's Milk Ice Cream is another option and easier to digest than cow dairy.

Fruit bowls
Combine sliced fruit and berries of choice with either some plain organic yogurt, goat's milk yogurt, coconut yogurt, or even eaten alone makes a great and healthy dessert. Recipe idea on next page.

Granola Bowls
Again you can use any fruits you like in their whole form, then sliced to bite size pieces, and stirred into granola or plain oats, and either eaten cold with Almond Milk or heated either in the oven or on the stove top in a saucepan and served warm. You choose.

Fruit Creation Bowl

What you will need:

1 Apple sliced into small cubes
1 Pear sliced into small cubes
1 Banana sliced
1 A handful of whole Strawberries sliced in half
1 A handful of Red and Green Grapes
1 A handful of Sliced Pineapple
½ Cup Whole Raspberries

Mixed with any yogurt of choice (from the previous page) and serve.
Or stir with grated ginger, 1 TBS maple syrup, and sprinkle with a little cinnamon and serve that way.
You can use any variation of fruits listed or use others that you enjoy.

In Closing

I hope you enjoyed learning a little bit about eating Holistically and finding new ways to incorporate it into your daily life. I also hope you enjoyed some recipes and are open to learn new ways to cook and eat so you feel your best in everything you do.

My Wish For You

May you try your best to shift into eating better and living a more fulfilling life.

May you find your way to health and wellness.

May you feel better and better every day as you choose what's good and right for you and your body.

May you be the best version of yourself in every way you can.

May you grow and evolve as you eat better and become more active.

May you find the life you were always meant to live.

May you love yourself and your body for the beautiful creation it is.

Blessings All.